Y0-ASJ-808

Improving Your Health with Vitamin E

by Ruth Adams
and
Frank Murray

Preventive Health
Library
Series

Larchmont Books
New York

First printing: June, 1978

IMPROVING YOUR HEALTH WITH VITAMIN E

Copyright © Larchmont Books, 1978

ISBN 0-915962-22-5

Printed in the United States of America

LARCHMONT BOOKS
*6 East 43rd Street
New York, N.Y. 10017
212-949-0800*

Contents

CHAPTER 1
The Importance of Vitamin E 5
CHAPTER 2
Yes, Vitamin E Is Safe 36
CHAPTER 3
Vitamin E and Heart Disease 48
CHAPTER 4
Vitamin E and Aging 68
CHAPTER 5
Vitamin E and Air Pollution 81
CHAPTER 6
Vitamin E Is Important for
a Successful Pregnancy 87
CHAPTER 7
What's Wrong When Healthy Babies
Suddenly Die 96
CHAPTER 8
Premature Babies and Vitamin E 108
CHAPTER 9
Vitamin E for Burns, Wounds, Bed
Sores and Scars 118
CHAPTER 10
Other Skin Disorders 124
CHAPTER 11
Varicose Veins 130
CHAPTER 12
Buerger's Disease 135
CHAPTER 13
Vitamin E for Gum Health 137

CHAPTER 14
Vitamin E and Selenium Are
Related 146
CHAPTER 15
Natural vs. Synthetic Vitamin E 155
CHAPTER 16
Food Technologists Assess
Vitamin E 159
Suggested Further Reading.................................... 163
Index... 164

CHAPTER 1

The Importance of Vitamin E

FOR MANY YEARS the official position on vitamin E was that no one knows how much of it is needed every day by a healthy adult. Thus, the official booklet, *Recommended Dietary Allowances*, stated that "it is difficult to make any recommendation other than that the tocopherol (vitamin E) requirement will vary between 10 and 30 milligrams a day for adults. . . . The estimated average daily adult consumption of vitamin E has been calculated to be about 14 milligrams."

In 1968, when the Food and Nutrition Board, National Academy of Sciences-National Research Council, issued the revised *Recommended Daily Dietary Allowances*, vitamin E requirements were given as 20 to 30 International Units (I.U.) for adult men and women. But the revised RDAs published in 1974 had lowered the average daily requirement to 12 to 15 I.U. for adults.

We will use the terms "milligrams" and "International Units" interchangeably throughout this book. For a fuller explanation, see pages 16, 157.

Of course, when the term "average daily consumption"

5

is used, we individuals are not taken into account. Averages are made up of figures both above and below a given level. If the "average" American is getting the originally suggested 14 milligrams of vitamin E a day, this means that millions of Americans are getting less than this. It depends on what they are eating. However, up to now, The Establishment has gone on the assumption that the average American is all they are concerned with and, since this mythical person is getting 14 milligrams of vitamin E a day, there is no need for him to get any additional vitamin E in foods like wheat germ, or in food supplements.

In its July, 1965 issue, *The American Journal of Clinical Nutrition* published an article by four drug company researchers who decided to find out exactly how much vitamin E there is in the average diet. They selected foods in a grocery store which might be typical, they thought, of the breakfasts, lunches and dinners we eat. Since salad oils contain considerable amounts of vitamin E, they included as many foods as possible that might be prepared with salad oils. They used margarine as well as butter. They used mayonnaise.

They planned menus for eight days which are much more nutritious than most Americans eat, we believe. With the increase of "junk" and convenience foods now on the market, we also believe that the American diet has declined even more since 1965.

At any rate, one breakfast planned by the researchers consisted of one-half cup of tomato juice, three-fourths cup of cooked wheat and barley cereal, two slices of whole wheat bread, two pats of margarine, two slices of ham, one egg, coffee and sugar, four ounces of milk for cereal and coffee. Do you know anybody who eats that much for breakfast?

A typical luncheon menu contained: three slices of liverwurst, two slices of whole wheat bread, seven leaves of lettuce, one medium tomato, one tablespoon of mayonnaise, one slice of pound cake (lots of butter in this), 1/6

6

quart of chocolate ice cream, and six ounces of milk.

Judging from all the surveys of peoples' eating habits that have been done by nutrition experts, very few people indeed eat as varied and plentiful a diet as this. Teenagers, we are told, eat scanty breakfasts, if any. Lunch for them may consist of a soft drink and potato chips, candy, etc. Older people tend to eat only cereals, sweets, tea and toast. Few people ever try purposely to plan meals with an eye specifically to their vitamin E content, as these researchers did.

Yet, in spite of the fact that these meals were planned especially for a high vitamin E content, the researchers found that they came to an overall daily average of only 7.4 milligrams of vitamin E, or just about one-half of the current recommended daily dietary allowance for the vitamin.

The scientists said that their research indicates the possibility of relatively low vitamin E intake in a portion of the population "depending somewhat on dietary habits." They added that "this observation points up the importance of doing more work in this area to establish more accurately the actual intake of both vitamin E and the unsaturated fats in order better to assess the adequacy of vitamin E in the 'average' American diet."

In the *New England Journal of Medicine* for December 9, 1965, a group of physicians reported that **of 55 patients with digestive complaints, 17 were deficient in vitamin E.** All of these folks had some evidence that they were not digesting food thoroughly. The researchers say that many of the symptoms of vitamin E deficiency are likely to be diagnosed as something else by doctors, so the condition may remain undiscovered.

And so we may become deficient in vitamin E because we are not eating vitamin E rich foods or we are not absorbing enough vitamin E from the foods we are eating. We shall soon see another reason why we may be short on vitamin E—the food may simply be grown with a low level

7

of the vitamin.

Our all-knowing Food and Drug Administration tells us in every press release attacking us "food faddists" that we are entirely incorrect when we say that the way food is raised or treated influences its nutritive content. No matter how the crop is fertilized, the FDA claims, no matter whether organic or chemical fertilizers are used, no matter whether the crop is grown on soil that has been depleted of much of its mineral wealth through years of farming, the vitamin and mineral content of the food will remain the same, according to the experts in Washington. So long as the soil is in good enough condition to produce a crop at all, the food produced will contain plenty of vitamins and minerals. Any further attention to fertilizers may produce a bigger crop, but the nutritive content will remain the same, the FDA experts say.

We health conscious folks have always contended that **many people in our country may be shortchanged in their nutrition program because their food has been grown on soil from which much of the nutritional value has been depleted**. Trace minerals, for instance, have been taken off in crop after crop and never replaced by fertilizers. The usual commercial fertilizer contains only three or four of the best known and most widely used minerals and ignores the trace elements. Organic gardening and farming assures an ample supply of these important elements by replacing in the soil all possible living matter: leaves, grass, clippings, hay, straw and animal products like bone meal, manure and so forth.

It is difficult, time-consuming and expensive to prove our point, for it involves testing foods from many different soils and growing conditions to determine their nutritive content. The experts in Washington can always belittle our tests by claiming that certain varieties of vegetables or grains have genetic ability to produce food high in certain vitamins and minerals. If we find a food high in a vitamin,

8

they will say that the organic gardening method wasn't responsible for its vitamin content—it's just that the gardener planted a certain variety of seed which produces a food high in that vitamin. In a 1973 press release the FDA reported that "levels naturally found in animal feed vary widely depending on the soil in which the feed crops were grown." The FDA estimated that approximately 70 per cent of American corn and soybeans do not contain sufficient selenium, the trace mineral.

We were interested, therefore, in looking through a very official book from the Agricultural Experiment Station at the University of Wyoming to find that **tests on food raised throughout the world showed an astonishing range in the content of one vitamin—vitamin E**. The book is entitled, *Vitamin E Content of Foods and Feeds for Human and Animal Consumption.*

For example, the vitamin E content of corn oil sold in the United States may vary from 79 milligrams in a given quantity of oil to as much as 239 milligrams of vitamin E. In other words, you may purchase one brand of corn oil which will give you three times more vitamin E than another brand. Cottonseed oil, a very popular salad oil, may contain 96 milligrams of vitamin E or as little as 53 milligrams. Both in the same bottles, perhaps the same brand.

Olive oil sold in the U. S. may contain as little as 6.9 milligrams of vitamin E or as much as 30 milligrams—almost five times more. Peanut oil may vary from 15 milligrams to 59 milligrams. Safflower oil may vary from 16.9 to 49.2 milligrams. Soybean oil may vary from 44 to 219 milligrams—five times as much. Crude wheat germ oil may contain 190 milligrams of vitamin E or up to 420 milligrams.

What about wheat? One sample of American wheat showed a total of only 0.03 milligram of vitamin E in a given quantity, while another sample contained 2.87

milligrams—90 times more than the first sample.

We confined our observations to American products. But looking at figures from other countries, we found many much wider variations in vitamin E content of foods.

The University of Wyoming book states, "Recent reports on the vitamin E content of blood from people in the United States and Great Britain show that **a small percentage of the population has dangerously low blood levels of vitamin E.**" Some people are making every effort to eat more foods that contain the unsaturated fats, trying to prevent cholesterol deposits in blood vessels. These fats raise one's requirement for vitamin E. That is, if you eat lots of the cereal and vegetable oils, you need to get lots of vitamin E as well.

So the vitamin E content of one's food is quite important. If one is depending on a corn oil for its vitamin E content, chances are that one will consistently buy the same brand of oil at the same store. Now if the corn oil company checks the vitamin E content of its products constantly, one may be getting about the same amount of this vitamin in every bottle. But the likelihood of a company's going to this trouble seems remote, especially since the vitamin E content of any salad oil does not have to be stated on the label.

In any case, no matter what it is that causes these immense differences in the nutritive content of foods we buy at the store, how can the FDA experts continue to say that we are all certain to get all the nutrition we need, no matter what brand we buy?

The mother who feeds her children bread made from one kind of American-grown wheat will be providing them with 90 times more vitamin E than another mother who buys bread made from another kind of wheat. Wheat is our best food source of vitamin E. Bleaching it to obtain white bread destroys much of its vitamin E content. So the child who eats white bread made from flour containing 0.03 milligram of vitamin E is getting almost no vitamin E, while the fortunate child who eats wholegrain bread made from a wheat containing 90 times more vitamin E to begin with, is getting 90 times more value from this important food.

Two researchers at Distillation Products Industries have measured the amount of vitamin E in grains of various kinds, and then have measured the vitamin E content of a number of products made from these grains. **The amount of vitamin E that is lost is appalling, and the evidence shows that the different kinds of processing result in differing amounts of loss**. It seems true, as well, that the more processing the food goes through, the greater the loss.

In the July-August, 1969 issue of *Agricultural and Food Chemistry*, Drs. David C. Herting and Emma-Jane E. Drury report that they obtained samples of grain from various parts of the United States. Corn came from seven states, wheat from six states, oats from three states and rice from three states. And they bought processed cereals and flours from local grocery stores.

They found, first, **that samples of the grain itself contained differing amounts of vitamin E depending, they believe, on the variety of grain planted, where it was grown, the time of harvest and the stability of the grain after harvesting**. One sample, for instance, had been stored for six years and showed a very low level of vitamin E even without any processing. Presumably the vitamin had disappeared during storage.

Then they compared the vitamin E content of each sample with a sample of some processed food containing the same grain. The results are very revealing. **In some cases up to 98 per cent of the vitamin was lost**. Losses for corn ranged from 35 per cent lost in processing white meal to 98 per cent for one kind of corn flakes. Wheat lost from 22 per cent for one puffed product cereal up to 92 per cent for one brand of flour. Interestingly enough, oatmeal showed almost no loss of vitamin E. But, as more extensive processing was done, almost all the vitamin E was lost from this cereal too. Rice cereals lost more than 70 per cent of

11

their vitamin E content.

Each brand of processed cereal showed different losses. Some had as much as five times the amount of vitamin E that others had. They do not know, say the authors, whether the loss results from removal of the vitamin, as when corn or wheat germ is removed, since most of the vitamin E is in the germ, or whether the processing creates a direct destruction of the vitamin. And nobody knows, they tell us, what happens to the remaining vitamin E after the product is put on the shelf. How much more of it disappears before it is eaten?

Another important aspect of this problem, as we have stated, is that **vitamin E is related to the amount of unsaturated fats in any food:** There should be a certain ratio or balance between these two nutrients. This is why we have been warned not to go overboard eating large amounts of the unsaturated fats without a considerable amount of vitamin E along with them. Now we find, due to processing, the ratio of these important fats and vitamin E may vary from a range of 0.10 all the way up to 1 in one sample of whole wheat. Processing which would remove almost all of the vitamin E might make for a very serious situation in regard to this important ratio in the final product.

The authors of the report on vitamin E suggest that the best thing to do is to fortify cereals with vitamin E to restore the amount lost in processing. They say that a researcher named Rubin and another named Harris recommended several years ago that refined, white flour be fortified with vitamin E and in 1969 another scientist proposed it for cereals. The authors agree.

Are you still convinced that you get plenty of vitamin E in your diet? Don't be too sure. Four British researchers undertook to measure the amount of vitamin E in the average British diet and reported their findings in the *British Journal of Nutrition*, Vol. 26: 89, 1971. **They found that most of the people studied have less than 5 milligrams**

12

a day of vitamin E.

The *Journal of the American Dietetic Association*, Vol. 63, page 147, 1973, reports on the amount of vitamin E in "the average American diet." **Of the diets studied, a low-fat, low-calorie breakfast contained only half a milligram of vitamin E**. The breakfast consisted of orange juice, toast, dry cereal and milk.

A high-fat, high-calorie dinner of tomato juice, calf liver and bacon, mashed potatoes, lima beans, spinach, roll with margarine, salad with dressing and cake had only 5.7 milligrams of vitamin E. Adding up a series of low-fat breakfasts, lunches and dinners, the authors found that they contained a total of only 4.4 milligrams of vitamin E. The high-fat, high-calorie breakfasts, lunches and dinners came to 12.7 milligrams per day. It thus appears that "typical" American diets may vary widely in their content of vitamin E—an average of about 8 milligrams a day.

In the August, 1974 issue of *The Journal of the American Geriatrics Society*, E. Cheraskin, M.D., D.M.D., W. M. Ringsdorf, Jr., D.M.D., and B. S. Hicks published an article, "Eating Habits of the Dentist and His Wife: Daily Consumption of Vitamin E." They tell us that they collected information from a group of 369 dentists and 288 wives on what they ate every day for one week. They kept very careful records, with special attention to the frequency with which they ate certain foods—in this case, foods in which there is lots of vitamin E.

The information was analyzed by a computer. The results were discussed with the people involved. They were told of the relationship between good nutrition and good health, especially, in this case, getting enough vitamin E. They were told how they could increase their intake of vitamin E and why they should.

About one year later, the survey was made again. Every participant kept account of every food eaten during one week. Similar surveys were taken every year for four years for the same group of people, so that the researchers now have a good idea of just what foods are eaten daily by each member of this group and how much vitamin E is contained in each day's diet.

At the same time, the same group of volunteers were being given certain tests to determine just what their condition was in regard to heart and circulatory health. Some of them showed improved health in this area. Others showed no improvement or little improvement. These facts were then correlated with the amounts of vitamin E which each individual got in his daily diet. It's hard to imagine a more comprehensive and convincing way to arrive at the facts.

One object was to see if those who had not been getting enough vitamin E would increase their intake after a period of nutritional education. Another object was to see if an increase in the amount of vitamin E in the daily diet would improve heart and circulatory health and if a decrease in the amount of vitamin E in the daily diet would cause lack of improvement or even a turn for the worse in heart and circulatory health.

The results are enlightening. **First of all, the Alabama scientists found that there was a wide range of vitamin E intake among the volunteer dentists and their wives.** Among the dentists, some got as little as 6 International Units of vitamin E daily, some as much as 212 units. Forty-six per cent of all the dentists got, at meals, less than 30 units daily, which was the recommended daily allowance until recently. Their wives also got widely varying amounts of vitamin E. Some got as little as 4 units, others as much as 213. Forty-five per cent of the wives were getting less than the 25 units daily which were until recently recommended by federal experts.

How did they do after the nutritional education course? The average amount of daily intake of vitamin E at the beginning of the test was 21 units in a selected group of 84 paired subjects. At the second visit, after the nutritional instruction, these same people were getting an average of 51 units. And at the third visit they were getting 127 units of the vitamin. So there is no doubt that a simple course of instruction in nutrition can improve the intake of nutrients among those who wish to show improvement. In other words, it's perfectly possible to learn how to get more of a given vitamin at meals, if you want to.

And what happened to the health of the people who arranged their eating patterns so that they got more vitamin E? You have perhaps guessed what happened. **As the intake of vitamin E went up, so did the heart and circulatory health improve**. When the intake went up only slightly there was little or no noticeable improvement. But when daily intake went up considerably, there was considerable improvement in circulatory conditions. This was determined, incidentally, by use of the Cornell Medical Index Questionnaire on which various facts in regard to heart and circulation are recorded.

The Alabama researchers report that the dose of vitamin E seems to be very important in regard to benefits received. **Dosages twice as high as those officially recommended appeared to be the most beneficial.**

Why is vitamin E so important to health? Well, there is an abundance of medical literature showing that **deficiency in vitamin E may be largely responsible for heart and artery disorders which are the number one killers in our period of history**. Vitamin E is essential for the health of muscles. Muscular diseases of mysterious origin plague hundreds of thousands. Vitamin E is essential for the health of the reproductive system. Complaints of infertility, miscarriage, menopause and menstruation disorders yield usually to large doses of vitamin E plus a diet that includes plenty of this nutrient. Don't believe that old saw that vitamin E is an aphrodisiac and thus will improve your love-life. But vitamin E does aid in increasing the sperm count and in correcting other errors of infertility.

Dr. Evan Shute of the Shute Foundation for Medical Research in London, Canada, summarizes the effects of vitamin E in human beings in the 1975 issue of *The Summary*, published by the Foundation. **Dr. Shute says that vitamin E does the following:**

Reduces oxygen requirements in tissues. Melts fresh blood clots by a process called fibrinolysis. Rapidly increases the extent of collateral circulation—that is, it builds auxiliary blood vessels around places which are blocked with blood clots. Dilates capillaries, the smallest of the blood vessels. Occasionally removes excessive scar tissue. Prevents overproduction of scar tissue. Prevents scar tissue contraction as wounds heal. Mobilizes and increases platelets. These are tiny blood cells. Is one of the regulators of fat and protein metabolism. The vitamin E should be natural and labeled in International Units. Natural vitamin E is called *d* alpha tocopherol to distinguish it from synthetic vitamin E, which is called *dl* alpha tocopherol (this is a lower case "L" and not the number "one").

Incidentally, the confusion over whether to speak of vitamin E in terms of milligrams or International Units arises from the fact that the international standard for alpha tocopherol was set using the synthetic form (dl). **One I.U. of dl-alpha tocopherol equals 1 milligram. But in the case of the "natural" vitamin E, 1 milligram equals 1.49 International Units.**

Throughout this book we have reported on many uses for vitamin E. We follow with some brief discussions about various applications.

Studying the condition of red blood cells in eight people, two British scientists gave them 200 milligrams of vitamin E daily by mouth and 100 milligrams by injection. Six of the patients had diseases which prevented them from absorbing vitamins. The two others were alcoholics on poor diets. The doctors found that these rather large doses of vitamin E greatly improved the health of the red blood cells. The research was reported in the *American Journal of Clinical Nutrition*, Vol. 24:388, 1971.

The sports editor of a Midwest newspaper reported in 1962 on the use of vitamin E and wheat germ oil by athletes. One runner, who was 64, ran a mile in five minutes, 30 seconds. **He attributed his stamina to vitamin E.** Another "miler" used wheat germ in his diet when he was breaking mile records. Swimmers and runners of international repute also use wheat germ. When American athletes were polled at the Olympic Games in Rome in 1960, it turned out that 88 per cent of them use wheat germ, 86 per cent use wheat germ oil and 84 per cent use vitamin preparations of some kind. Some use all three.

As the Soviet Academy of Medical Sciences announced they had found vitamin E very helpful to Russian athletes, a New Jersey physician asked some searching questions about the possibility of harm to future generations in the steroid drugs taken by many athletes in this country.

Said *Medical Tribune* for April 12, 1972: **"Supplementary vitamin E improves the performance capacity of such sportsmen as skiers and racing cyclists,** according to investigators at the Soviet Academy of Medical Sciences Nutrition Institute and the Central Institute of Physical Culture."

The Russian specialists carried out a three-week study of 34 cyclists and 37 skiers to determine, if possible, the vitamin E requirements under training and competition conditions. The athletes were divided into groups and each group was given a different amount of vitamin E. Those who got no extra vitamin E were getting about 15 to 20 milligrams of vitamin E in their food.

The athletes who got no additional vitamin E showed lower levels of the vitamin during the training period, indicating that the vitamin is used up during this time. In those men who got an additional 50 to 300 milligrams of vitamin E, the levels of the vitamin in the blood remained normal or were increased.

The Russian doctors found that the addition of 100 to 150 I.U. of vitamin E daily was best for a training period of

17

three to four hours.

One would imagine, on the basis of this information and the wealth of material in medical journals on the importance of vitamin E for athletic performance, that coaches and trainers of American sports performers would rush to buy the vitamin and give it to their teams. Instead, according to Dr. Max M. Novich of New Jersey, American athletes in some sports almost universally take steroid drugs to increase their weight and presumably their strength. They do this even though repeated tests have shown no improvement in strength, performance or work capacity. Apparently, the weight gain, valued by football players, weight lifters, basketball players and track athletes, is brought on by accumulations of fluid or just plain overeating.

If taken in heavy doses or over long periods of time, said Dr. Novich, "these drugs could produce very serious sexual difficulties, or may render the athletes impotent. Of all the drugs used by athletes," said Dr. Novich, "I find this the most disquieting because it works so subtly. Steroid use when not indicated is bad business."

Two American physicians, reporting in *Clinical Research* in 1963, discussed a patient of 46 who showed "progressive muscular weakness" for four years. **Giving him 300 milligrams of vitamin E daily produced a slow but striking improvement**. After 12 weeks therapy was stopped and soon the troubles began again. The condition of this man's muscles closely resembled that of rabbits deficient in vitamin E, say these physicians.

Two Japanese physicians reported in *Medical World News* in 1966 that they found **arthritis patients could take hormone drugs for their disorder with fewer side effects when they were also given 150 to 600 milligrams of vitamin E daily**. The authors believe that the vitamin might be used to prevent the bone-softening effect that these drugs often produce.

Dental Abstracts for September, 1973 tells of 14 patients

with gum (periodontal) disease. They were given 800 milligrams of vitamin E daily. **The vitamin reduced inflammation after 21 days**, so it should help to prevent bone loss in the jaw.

In an issue of *The Summary*, a Long Island, New York doctor tells **the almost unbelievable story of 20 schizophrenic patients at a mental hospital** suffering from complications of circulatory troubles in their legs and feet. One had a perforating ulcer which had not healed in two years. Nine others had skin disorders over both legs. All of them were diabetic; three had gangrene.

The doctor started them on 20 capsules daily of vitamin E (400 units per capsule). Later he raised the dosage to 40 capsules daily. The gangrene healed. The patient with the ulcer no longer must wear orthopedic shoes because of the sore. The patients went on to take 20 capsules daily of 400 units of vitamin E. For four months after the healing they are well and without leg pains. The doctor who performed this near-miracle is Dr. A. J. DeLiz. He stated that internists who visited and observed these changes described them as "incredible."

An Italian medical journal described the results of treatment of "bed sores" in rats. "Decubitus ulcers" is the way the doctors name them. The ulcers developed in five weeks and went on for up to five months. Each animal was then given 65 milligrams of vitamin E daily—an immense dose for so small an animal. Fifteen animals were not given the vitamin, so they acted as "controls." Within two weeks the ulcers healed in those animals which got the vitamin E.

In a Hungarian medical journal, Dr. F. Gerloczy tells of the **beneficial effects of vitamin E on a number of people suffering from various circulatory disorders**. He gave the vitamin in enormous doses—up to 24,000 milligrams or units daily. In some diseases "spectacular" results were obtained: in 10 cases of thrombosis of the arteries, 16 cases of thrombophlebitis, and 12 out of 15 cases of thromboangiitis obliterans (Buerger's Disease). In other cases of circulatory troubles, the doctor reported great relief in some patients, little improvement in others. One patient who had had a leg ulcer for 20 years was healed completely after only six weeks on vitamin therapy internally, plus vitamin E ointment on the skin.

Three Italian physicians used vitamin E to treat complications of hardening of the arteries in old folks. They were suffering from the mental symptoms that sometimes accompany this disease: confusion, loss of memory, dizziness, and generally decreased mental acuteness. Forty eight patients were given six capsules of vitamin E daily. The capsule contained 150 milligrams of vitamin E. **Improvement occurred, measured by memory, general intellectual status and other evidence of deficient circulation to the brain**. Associative memory showed the greatest improvement. Dizziness responded in some cases. All the patients became livelier and more talkative. The doctors plan longer trials and larger doses.

Intermittent claudication is a circulatory disorder of the legs and feet which makes it almost impossible to walk any distance because of the extreme pain. A Swedish physician wrote in a Swedish medical journal in 1973 on his study of 47 patients. All suffered from a closing off of the leg circulation due to **hardening of the arteries**. The doctor gave them 300 units of vitamin E daily and instructed them to exercise as much as possible and to walk daily. **There was significant improvement within four to six months**.

In a similar group of patients who did not take vitamin E, two patients had to have their legs amputated, since the disease had progressed so far. After two years of treatment with vitamin E, the flow of blood through the legs of other patients was greatly improved. The doctor believes that the pain of intermittent claudication is not caused just by the lack of circulation, but by the muscle degeneration which follows.

Seven Canadian scientists reported in the *Canadian Journal of Physiology and Pharmacology* (3:384, 1974) that, in pregnancies ending in still births, the vitamin E content of blood was lower than in normal pregnancies. Studies in animals indicated that a mother who is deficient in vitamin E is more likely to have congenital malformations in her offspring. The authors suggest that "the possibility of a vitamin basis for congenital deformities may be worth testing."

Another group of Canadian doctors studied the vitamin E status of people with various thyroid disorders and reported their findings in the *Journal of Canadian Medical Women's Association*. They found, they said, that vitamin E levels were low in the blood of people whose thyroid glands were overactive. An overactive thyroid gland can result in gross underweight, nervousness, bulging eyes and fast heart beat.

Federation Proceedings, July-August, 1965, which we reviewed, reported that a diet deficient in vitamin E causes the body to be unable to use all its methionine, which is one of the important amino acids or forms of protein. The brain, muscles, heart and kidneys suffered as a result. And the diet being eaten was completely nourishing except for lack of vitamin E.

In a fascinating letter to the editor of *Archives of Dermatology*, Vol. 108, page 855, 1973, two physicians report using vitamin E for patients suffering from neuralgia which afflicted them after a session of shingles (herpes). The doctors treated 13 patients with oral and topical vitamin E. That is, they gave them vitamin E by mouth and used the ointment on the affected skin. Eleven of these patients had suffered more than six months, seven for more than one year, one for 13 years and one for 19 years. These two last patients had almost complete relief from pain with the vitamin E treatment. Two were moderately improved and two were slightly improved. The doctors gave dosages of 400 to 1,600 units of vitamin E per day.

One of these patients had angina (the agonizing chest pain that afflicts heart patients). Taking 1,200 units of

vitamin E daily, she controlled the neuralgia. She also cured the leg cramps she had suffered from and found that she no longer needed nitroglycerin, the drug she had been taking to control the angina.

Quokkas are nocturnal wallabies, little animals from Australia about the size of rabbits, which have been imported into this country for investigations at the University of Cincinnati Medical Center. It seems the quokkas often develop progressive muscular weakness when they are fed diets deficient in vitamin E. Giving them supplements of the vitamin completely reverses the condition. The muscle difficulties of these and other animals and birds are quite related, it seems, to human diseases involving muscles, including muscular dystrophy. With tools and machinery of unimaginable complexity, scientists at the Center will try to discover more about the nutritional aspects of this class of muscle diseases— including vitamin E.

A vitamin E deficiency causes muscular dystrophy in monkeys. Lack of the vitamin causes the accumulation of cholesterol in muscles with the crippling effects of dystrophy. Dr. Manford D. Morris of the University of Arkansas, who is working with dystrophic monkeys, stated in 1968 that vitamin E deficiency cannot be the cause of MD in human beings, because "such deficiency in humans is extremely rare, and probably non-existent in the United States." It seems he has not read the surveys showing that vitamin E deficiency may, instead, be very common among Americans.

The Australian Veterinarian, Vol. 46:405, 1970 tells of a number of cattle dying of muscular dystrophy. They were being transported on shipboard. They died overnight. Their blood showed the usual levels of vitamin E and selenium, a mineral which is closely related to vitamin E in function.

To see if they could prevent such a tragedy from happening again, the vets in charge on the next trip gave the cattle selenium and vitamin E. The selenium alone did not help. But giving vitamin E with the mineral prevented any deaths from MD among the animals.

In *Veterinary Medicine*, Vol. 66:500, 1971, an American scientist, J. B. Herrick, reports on these animal diseases which can be cured by giving vitamin E: muscular dystrophy in cattle, sheep, swine and poultry; encephalomalacia and exudative diathesis in poultry; liver necrosis in swine; impaired reproduction and birth defects in several species; enlarged hock disorder in chickens and turkeys.

In the June 6, 1977 issue of *Chemical and Engineering News*, we learn that **vitamin E reduces the heart damage** associated with the anticancer drug adriamycin in laboratory mice, according to scientists at the National Cancer Institute. This drug is used to treat at least 10 kinds of human cancer, but its effects on the heart may be so severe that its use may be limited. It may cause congestive heart failure.

The experiment came about partly because of earlier work that had shown that the cancer drug produces a certain substance in the blood which vitamin E can completely block. The substance apparently releases "free radicals" which are toxic substances. Vitamin E scavenges such chemicals—that is, just envelopes them and renders them harmless.

So the group of NCI researchers gave their laboratory mice 85 units of vitamin E 24 hours before they gave them a dose of the cancer drug. A second group received the cancer drug without any vitamin E. Within one month 85 per cent of the mice which had received no vitamin E were dead, while 85 per cent of the mice that had gotten the vitamin E were still alive and healthy. Synthetic chemicals which can supposedly destroy free radicals were also tried and had no helpful effect on the mice treated with the cancer drug.

Examining the hearts of the mice, the scientists found absolutely no damage to the heart muscle in the mice which got the vitamin E, while those which did not get the vitamin

E had extensive damage. Vitamin E also appeared to prevent the damage to liver and duodenum which was apparent in those mice which got no vitamin.

And how did vitamin E affect the drug's action on the cancer? It had little if any detrimental effect. In 60 animals in whom cancers had been implanted, those previously treated with vitamin E lived considerably longer than untreated mice. The scientists also believe that when vitamin E is given previously the animals can safely be given larger doses of the cancer drug.

The NCI scientists said they were not sure if their findings could be applied to human beings with cancer. Human cancers differ from animal cancers, they said. And human tumors differ from one another in their reactions. It's probable, they said, that the amount of vitamin E which they gave the mice, translated into dosages suitable for human beings, might not be absorbed from the digestive tract. We don't know why the NCI scientists say this, since there seems to be no evidence that the average person has any difficulty in absorbing this vitamin from the digestive tract.

According to two Japanese physicians, **vitamin E gives valuable assistance to patients who are being treated with hormones**, sometimes called "steroids." These powerful drugs, which alleviate symptoms of pain and swelling, also produce such extremely serious side effects that often they must be discontinued. But when vitamin E in quite large doses is given with them, side effects are eliminated and eventually the doses of the powerful drugs can be reduced or stopped.

The two Kyoto Medical College professors used from 150 to 600 milligrams of vitamin E daily. They tell the story of one 29-year-old housewife who had rheumatism of the elbows, arms, fingers and legs. Her condition was deteriorating with very high doses of the steroids. And when the doctors tried to reduce the dosage, she returned to the clinic, barely able to walk.

24

At this point they gave her vitamin E along with the drugs. Seven months later she was discharged on a very small dose of the drug, plus vitamin E. At present, they say, she is "progressing." "She is able to enjoy folk dancing and bicycle riding."

The Japanese doctors also reported that other conditions related to blood vessels appear to be greatly improved when vitamin E is given. The vitamin appears to stimulate the circulation in the feet, legs and hands, they say. Furthermore the vitamin increases the flow of blood in both arteries and veins. Rheumatic patients report that they lose the "cold feeling" in their legs when they are on high doses of vitamin E. The vitamin seems to prevent blood vessels from becoming fragile and to increase the resistance in the walls of the tiny capillaries—the smallest of the blood vessels.

The two Japanese physicians discovered these properties of vitamin E when they treated a patient whose hand had been crushed beneath a great weight. Six months later a circulatory disturbance developed and the fingers began to turn blue and become very painful. The doctors gave large doses of vitamin E. After four months there was great improvement. Then they decided to try vitamin E on their rheumatic patients with the excellent results reported above. The information about this research was contained in an address before the Japanese Rheumatism Society. It was reported in the U.S. in *Medical World News*, July 1, 1966.

Cooley's Anemia is the name given to an inherited disease also called Mediterranean anemia or thalassemia major. It is most common among Italians and Greeks. Because of migration from these countries to the United States, it is becoming increasingly common in this country. The disease, caused by a mutation, may affect one child in every four born to parents both of whom carry the defective gene. Victims must have many blood transfusions, since they cannot manufacture healthy red blood cells.

The *British Journal of Hematology*, February, 1974, carried an article revealing a very low level of vitamin E in the blood of children with this disease who were receiving inadequate treatment with transfusions. **Giving them 200 milligrams of vitamin E daily improved the situation in six of the 21 children tested**. This does not mean that lack of the vitamin is a cause of the disease. But it certainly indicates the urgent need to do much more research on the possible relation of vitamin deficiency to this disorder and the possible amelioration of some of its manifestations which might be achieved by giving the vitamin in large doses.

"The September 20 news report on the effects of vitamin E on aging confirms what many of us have suspected for quite some time," reported Herbert Schwartz, Professor of Organic Chemistry, Cumberland County College, Vineland, New Jersey, in a letter to the editor of *The New York Times*, October 5, 1974.

"Since **vitamin E is destroyed by oxidants** (for it is an antioxidant), it can perform its service to the organism only while the supply lasts. Accordingly, an environment full of oxidants, e.g., ozone, nitrogen oxides, halogens, would deplete the stock of vitamin E in an organism, leading to premature aging.

"This line of reasoning would seem to confirm the observation that people in the cities seem to age faster than people in the country and that Americans seem to age faster than the people abroad. Could this be blamed upon the American habit of adding a soluble oxidant to the drinking water—namely chlorine?"

A bout of shingles is one of the most painful experiences anyone can have. It goes by the medical name of *herpes zoster*. It is caused by a virus, in the same family as the virus which causes cold sores. The pain follows the affected nerve right down across the body. Potent pain killers are necessary to ease it so that the patient can get through each day.

Now a group of Japanese doctors, writing in the Japanese medical journal, *Rinsho Derma*, 17:545, 1975 tell us they had **success treating the neuralgic pain with vitamin E**. They gave the vitamin (in large doses, we assume, although no mention is made of the dosage) to nine patients, of whom seven had excellent results, freeing them of pain in 14 and 21 days with "only slight anesthesia."

In a letter to The Shute Foundation, these same doctors from Sapporo tell of 28 patients suffering from the neuralgia related to shingles and 111 shingles patients who also got relief from vitamin E.

These doctors believe, they say, that getting oxygen to the painful spot may be the method by which vitamin E relieves the pain. They suggest that vitamin E might be used in other forms of neuralgia.

"Minamata Disease" is caused by mercury poisoning. It occurred sometime ago throughout an entire locality in Japan where a factory had been dumping mercurial waste in a lake from which the people of Minamata got their fish. Nerve cells were affected, resulting in devastating paralysis, brain damage, mental retardation, loss of hearing, speech and sight. Children born to women exposed to the mercury came into the world damaged for life.

A Japanese scientist reported in *Toxicology and Applied Pharmacology*, 32:347, 1975 that he believes **vitamin E may have the potential of rendering toxic mercury compounds less toxic**. He recounted only observations from his laboratory work. There was no attempt to give the vitamin as a protective or curative measure to anyone exposed to mercury. But his reasoning sounded good to doctors at the Shute Foundation.

A. Hoffer and R. M. Roy wrote in *Radiation Research*, 61:439, 1975 on the effects of **vitamin E in preventing damage from radiation**. Two groups of laboratory mice were irradiated. One group was given vitamin E. The other was not. Then the condition of their red blood cells was studied.

27

After exposure to high level radiation, the mice not protected by the vitamin E had red blood cells completely destroyed by the radiation. The red blood cells of those mice protected by vitamin E remained intact. The effect of radiation on blood cells has been studied in test tubes, say these two authors, but now we have firm evidence that the same protection is available in the living organism.

This suggests that anyone who is getting radiation treatment needs vitamin E to protect red blood cells. All of us are getting some radiation in everyday life, from background radiation and X-rays as well as the many radioactive substances released from bombs and nuclear power plants. So isn't it a good idea to get enough vitamin E for this reason alone, let alone all those other aspects of health which involve this very versatile vitamin?

"Whenever there is tissue injury—from a severe accident, extensive operation or destruction of tissue by cancer or infection—alterations in the constituents of blood occur which favor blood clotting," says Dr. Alton Ochsner, Professor Emeritus of Surgery at Tulane University School of Medicine. The body at all times responds to this kind of injury by activating its mechanism for clotting blood so that we do not bleed to death. So there is special danger from blood clots after major surgery.

In addition, the patient is lying quietly in bed. Blood in the veins of the legs is normally moved along and returned to the heart chiefly by the action of leg muscles, especially calf muscles. So lying quietly in bed without moving these muscles invites stagnation of the blood in veins. This is the main reason why it is now usual procedure to get surgery patients on their feet as soon as possible after operations. But we should also keep this consideration in mind when other illnesses or accidents confine us to bed. Blood clots are likely to form in our legs and move without warning into heart and/or lungs possibly causing death.

This condition is called phlebothrombosis. In 1948, a colleague of Dr. Ochsner's at Tulane discovered that

vitamin E, in the presence of calcium, decreased the incidence of clotting in a test tube. The vitamin was then given to patients at the medical center there who had severe injuries, hence were candidates for fatal blood clots. The incidence of these clots decreased decidedly. "It is for that reason that I have been using alpha tocopherol (vitamin E) since that time and have become very enthusiastic about its use in the prevention of intravenous clotting," says Dr. Ochsner in *Executive Health*, Vol. X, No. 5, 1974.

He also uses this vitamin for long-term prevention of unhealthful clotting, since it carries none of the hazards of anti-coagulant drugs. These drugs, unless monitored constantly, can cause hemorrhaging which can, of course, be fatal. Vitamin E does not produce this tendency in the blood.

Dr. Ochsner tells the story of a 43-year-old man whose blood indicated a tendency to clot. He developed pain in his right knee and hip along with a condition usually caused by a clot in the blood vessel of that region. The doctors decided to operate and replace the hip—an extremely serious operation. They gave the patient 200 units of vitamin E three times daily, then 100 units of vitamin E three times daily until they brought the clotting condition of his blood back to normal. Then they performed the operation, giving him more vitamin E after the operation. He recovered with no complications.

"I am convinced that its (vitamin E) use is extremely beneficial and at times life-saving," says Dr. Ochsner.

Dr. Ochsner also says that **vitamin C is helpful before and after surgery**. It, too, helps to control clotting in veins. He refers to a British experiment in which 30 of 63 surgery patients were given 1 gram (1,000 milligrams) of vitamin C daily before and after their operations. These were people up to the age of 84 undergoing very serious operations. Of the 30 patients given the vitamin C, only 10 had positive tests for clots, none had trouble in both legs and one had pulmonary clot. Of the 33 patients who were not given vitamin C, 20 (60 per cent) had positive tests for clots, in 10 of them both legs were involved and 12 patients had pulmonary clots. A most convincing bit of evidence.

Vitamin C, says Dr. Ochsner, is absolutely necessary for proper healing of wounds and by wounds he also means infections of any kind, for all infections cause injury to tissues. He describes a patient with extensive cancer of the jaw. Dr. Ochsner removed the malignant tissue but the wound did not heal. Instead it became infected. This was before the days of antibiotics. He gave the patient large doses of vitamin C, which controlled the infection and healed the wound.

In the January 10, 1972 issue of *The Journal of the American Medical Association*, Dr. Robert F. Cathcart III of Incline Village, Nev. says, "The increasing interest in vitamin E in California has led to tremendous public self-experimentation...." He refers to an article which appeared in a California medical journal where vitamin E in large doses was used successfully for leg cramps and for a condition called "restless legs." He tells us that such symptoms are common among his patients. **He began to prescribe vitamin E in doses of 300 units a day, first to patients with leg cramps, then to those complaining of pain in the neck and lower back**.

"I would agree," he says, "...that the medication is almost universally effective on...nocturnal leg cramps. In my opinion it is far more effective and safer to use than quinine or quinine-aminophylline combinations. Certainly the dosage we have been prescribing and the dosages taken (by health food advocates) are in excess of anything conceived of being a minimum daily requirement for the vitamin. The amount used is also far in excess of what could possibly be obtained through any reasonable normal diet."

He goes on to say that some patients who stop taking vitamin E are bothered by leg cramps in excess of those they first complained of. But only for a few days. After that, they disappear. It seems that leg cramps come and go among the folks that have them, so some people prefer to continue with the vitamin E doses while others use them just "over a crisis."

He says that other physicians have warned against using vitamin E with patients who have high blood pressure or diabetes. We would point out that Dr. Evan Shute says that patients with some kinds of high blood pressure may find that their pressure rises when they begin to take massive doses of vitamin E. So he suggests that they begin with quite small doses and increase them gradually. The same is true of some diabetics. Other diabetics find they can avoid many of the circulatory troubles that usually accompany this disease, if they take plenty of vitamin E daily.

Dr. Cathcart tells us that some of his patients find their leg cramps begin again if they decrease the dosage to 100 units daily. Others have found, after several months, that they must increase a dosage of 200 units daily to prevent symptoms. The physician says no one has needed more than 300 units. "I would second Ayres and Mihan's observations that massive doses of (vitamin E) are extremely effective in the control of idiopathic leg night cramps."

In another letter in the same issue of the *JAMA*, Dr. Samuel Ayres, Jr. of Los Angeles, describes his experience with 26 patients who suffered from leg cramps at night—"restless legs" and rectal cramps. **All of them obtained relief, he says, with doses of vitamin E ranging from 300 to 400 units daily, and sometimes as high as 800 units**.

He says he has written an article for publication documenting 76 cases "with equally good results." Some of these were "restless legs" cases, others had rectal cramps, and one young athlete training for the Olympics had severe cramps following strenuous exercise, including long-distance running, swimming and weight-lifting. "All of these patients received prompt and gratifying relief from the oral administration of vitamin E."

31

"I have to eat crow," said M. K. Horwitt, Professor of Biochemistry at St. Louis University School of Medicine, at a symposium on vitamin E. He was wrong about vitamin E all these years, he went on, for he has been saying what lots of establishment researchers have been saying—that we all get plenty of vitamin E in our meals and there's no reason to add more in the form of a supplement.

But Dr. Horwitt's more recent investigations have turned up such startling facts that **he is now recommending up to 800 units of vitamin E as insurance against the blood clots which complicate the lives of heart and circulatory patients**. Because of its effect on clotting, some doctors have been recommending large doses of aspirin to their patients, since aspirin is known to affect blood clotting. But vitamin E appears to be a better solution, said Dr. Horwitt.

Vitamin E breaks down in the body into a substance called d-alpha-tocopherol-quinone, which cancels out the work of vitamin K. Vitamin K is busy persuading the blood to coagulate, since this is its role in the body. But, in the case of heart attack victims (or, presumably people who may face such an emergency), the vitamin K is doing too good a job. The blood coagulates too readily.

In Sweden, said Dr. Horwitt, at a symposium of the Vitamin Information Bureau, **they tested nine patients who had had heart attacks. Doctors gave them 300 units of vitamin E daily. Within six weeks their "clotting time" tests showed improvement**. That is, the chances a blood clot would cause a stroke or heart attack were much less. Support for these Swedish researchers has recently appeared from a coagulation research group in this country, he went on.

Another drug often given to heart patients to prevent blood clots from forming is warfarin. This is effective because it destroys some vitamin K, thus preventing blood clots. But it must be given with great care and frequent blood tests must be taken, for a bit of an overdose can be so effective that hemorrhages take place, since the blood has been "thinned" too much. Strokes can result.

When doctors give warfarin and vitamin E at the same time, the vitamin E makes the drug more powerful so that even less time is needed to get the blood in such a condition that it will not clot. Laboratory scientists have found that rats, too, react this same way. Animals given warfarin show slower blood clotting if they are given, at the same time, either vitamin A, vitamin D or vitamin E.

So Dr. Horwitt recommends that, if doctors give vitamin E while they are giving warfarin or other anti-coagulants, they should decrease the dosage of the drug. It seems obvious, doesn't it, throughout all this discussion, although Dr. Horwitt does not mention it, that the body is trying to tell us that by correctly balancing all essential nutrients—like vitamin A, vitamin D and vitamin E—we need never have to take any drugs! The vitamins themselves will perform their duties of preventing clots from forming (vitamins A, D and E) or protecting the clotting ability of the blood so that we do not bleed to death. And this is the function of vitamin K.

What throws the whole mechanism out of kilter is the catastrophic imbalances created in modern diets when all the vitamin E is removed from the cereal foods that make up perhaps one-fourth of the avearage diet. And it is never returned. Nor do most of us ever get enough vitamin A to take care of all the functions of that essential nutrient. Human beings originated in the tropics where they got lots of sunshine on their bare skin the year around. The sunshine is converted into vitamin D in the body.

Dr. Horwitt urged doctors to consider vitamin E rather than other anti-coagulants. He also revealed that recent research has found that, in minor deficiencies of vitamin E, certain red blood cells are destroyed eight to 10 times faster than they should be. These cells are easily examined and tested, he said. But what about other body cells which doctors can't get at to test? Isn't it likely that the same premature destruction is also affecting them?

Another distinguished researcher at the same meeting, Dr. Daniel B. Menzel of Duke University, presented once again the compelling evidence of **vitamin E's protective action against certain elements in air pollution**. Certain kinds of fat in the lungs are destroyed by ozone and nitrogen oxide, both common ever-present air pollutants in urban localities. Testing lung cells exposed to these pollutants, Dr. Menzel found that 200 milligrams of vitamin E protected these cells against damage.

Then he tested the animals themselves. "Animals deficient in vitamin E died on an average 11.1 days after exposure to one part per million of ozone, while vitamin E supplemented animals died at 17 days," he said. Deficient animals exposed to 33 ppm of nitrogen oxide died after 8.2 days. Animals getting plenty of vitamin E averaged 18.5 days of life—more than twice as long.

He attributed these facts to the vitamin's ability to interfere with the oxidation, or destruction, of natural unsaturated fats in the lungs. Exposure to ozone causes lung cells to become viscous, he said, causing emphysema in the lungs—or cancer in other parts of the body. Getting enough vitamin E can prevent this damage.

Testing 11 human beings, Dr. Menzel found that diets containing 9 milligrams of vitamin E brought destruction to certain red blood cells. **After only one week of getting 100 milligrams of vitamin E, this damage disappeared**. The cells' resistance to damage was greatly increased, he said, when they were given 200 milligrams of vitamin E daily, and they continued to improve.

"The present dietary intake of vitamin E is inadequate to provide maximal protection against ozonides (ozone)," he said. He added that vitamin E supplementation might be beneficial in cases of pulmonary hypertension (high blood pressure), vascular (circulatory) disease, pulmonary embolism (a clot in the lungs) and disseminating vascular coagulation—that is, many blood clots in various parts of the body.

And so in reviewing some of the literature on vitamin E, we hope that we have convinced you of the importance of this vitamin, not only in possibly preventing an illness, but also in hopefully alleviating symptoms if you should develop certain disorders. In the following chapters we give you even more persuasive evidence of the importance and versatility of vitamin E.

CHAPTER 2

Yes, Vitamin E
Is Safe

IN RESPONSE TO what they called "the development of an apparent fad for vitamin E supplementation over the past few years," several researchers at the National Institutes of Health decided several years ago to find out just how harmful or harmless it might be to take large doses of vitamin E every day over a long period of time. A report on the results of this study appeared in the *American Journal of Clinical Nutrition* for December, 1975.

The two NIH scientists, Philip M. Farrell, M.D., Ph.D., and John G. Gieri, Ph.D., placed an ad in the local NIH newsletter. They asked for volunteers among people who had been taking large amounts of vitamin E for an average of three years or so.

They deliberately worded the ad to indicate that they were looking for "possible ill effects" so that no one would think they planned to promote the taking of vitamin E. They also wanted to be sure they would get enough volunteers for the survey.

Within one week they had 47 volunteers who had been taking from 100 to 1,000 International Units of the vitamin daily. Of these, 32 were selected for the study and 28 actually came in for the examinations.

Each was given a detailed four-page questionnaire about general health, and some questions about specific areas of health. Then the doctors took a complete medical history of each volunteer's past life. They took blood samples and tested them for many things. One question on the questionnaire inquired whether the volunteer had noted any difference in general health since taking vitamin E.

The ages of the volunteers ranged from 24 to 67. The general health of 22 of them was good. Six of them were going to doctors for one complaint or another. Nine volunteers took 100 to 200 units of vitamin E daily. Thirteen took 400 units and six took from 600 to 800 units. All but one of the volunteers also took other supplemental vitamins. Some of the volunteers had been taking vitamin E up to 21 years.

To decide whether the vitamin E had done any harm to any of the volunteers, 20 biochemical and blood tests were done—the same kinds of tests your doctor gives you. Six hundred tests in all were done for liver function, kidneys, thyroid gland, nerves, muscles and blood. Of the 600 tests, only seven abnormal results were found. One case was that of a volunteer taking a thyroid drug, whose thyroid hormone level was found to be high. Three volunteers showed high levels of triglycerides in the blood. Several others had minor discrepancies.

"On the basis of 20 laboratory screening tests per individual designed to assess a wide range of organ functions, it must be concluded that no signs of toxicity were uncovered in this investigation," say the two researchers who conducted the tests.

Half of the volunteers said they had noted improvement in health since taking vitamin E. Some noted smoother, clearer skin; two noted improvement in leg cramps; one had fewer headaches; one had fewer allergy symptoms; one had just general better health and several said that vitamin E had given them more energy.

"It is of interest to note," says the report, "that all subjects evaluated in this study began taking vitamin E on their own accord without a physician's recommendation. The majority commenced tocopherol (vitamin E) supplementation after reading about the vitamin in popular treatises. The dosages consumed under these voluntary conditions are, on the average, 30 times the recommended daily allowance."

The authors of the report do not want the professional readers of their material to get the idea that there may be scientific reference material available demonstrating the usefulness of vitamin E in a number of serious disorders, so they carefully state that, "Although proven tocopherol (vitamin E) deficiency in the absence of malabsorption is rare in this country, the popular press had proclaimed the vitamin as a prophylactic agent useful in cardiovascular disorders, intermittent claudication, diabetes mellitus, infertility, inflammatory skin diseases, pyorrhea and numerous other maladies."

They neglect to mention the many, many professional articles on these subjects which have appeared in authoritative medical and scientific journals from which, of course, the "popular press" has taken up the story. We review many of these articles in this book. They neglect to mention the many physicians and biochemists here and abroad who regularly use vitamin E for prevention and treatment of these conditions and for further experimentation in laboratories.

In any case, here is official reassurance from the very seat of the health establishment of the federal government—the National Institutes of Health—**that vitamin E in doses up to 800 milligrams daily has no deleterious effects on people who take the vitamin on their own**, without reference to any opinion their doctors may have or any other treatment their doctors may be giving them.

For those of you who may have hesitated to take large

doses of this vitamin, the research reported here seems reassuring. There is no reason to expect miracles. Those conditions for which treatment with vitamin E seems most effective have usually been building up for many years. They cannot be overcome in a matter of weeks or months. Vitamins don't "work" like drugs do, with an overnight sensational alleviation of whatever is wrong, followed by side effects that are often worse than the original complaint. Vitamins "work" with other vitamins and other nutrients to improve health generally and bring gradual but totally harmless benefit to conditions of ill health that may have prevailed for many years.

A letter to the editor of the *Toronto Star* from a Canadian physician is reproduced in a recent issue of *The Summary*, which is the publication of the Shute Institute in London, Ontario, Canada. In his letter, Dr. J. H. Barker is protesting a syndicated nutrition column which claimed that all of us get enough vitamin E in our meals, so we need not take additional amounts in supplements.

We've made a lot of serious errors about vitamin E, says Dr. Barker. For example, it was not until 1959 that vitamin E was declared officially to be essential for human health. Only in 1968 were we told how much we need every day—a maximum of 30 units for an adult. But nutritionists immediately began to complain that they could not possibly plan meals which would contain this much vitamin E daily. So—always eager to placate the nutritional establishment—the "experts" in Washington lowered the daily requirement to 15 units.

All the experts have known for years that the average American diet does not contain 30 milligrams daily, so by reducing the recommended daily amount to 15 milligrams the experts could presumably feel safer about the whole thing. Also, they figured, if they lowered the daily recommended amount, they might not draw so much flak from people in and out of university biology departments who keep insisting that vitamin E is almost totally lacking in the American diet, and that it becomes more and more essential every day as heart and circulatory conditions become more prevalent.

Says Dr. Barker, "The above figures were influenced by two erroneous concepts and one large hang-up. The first dubious concept is that one can obtain really reliable information about the amount of stored vitamin reserves in our body by measuring the level of vitamin in the blood plasma, an idea which has been challenged for a quarter century, but which still dominates our thinking. The second faulty and very dangerous assumption is that in the absence of obvious signs of vitamin deficiency in the population, the diet must therefore be adequate. That is, one just measures the amount of vitamin E in the diet, and that must be the amount we require. However, optimal health is clearly more than the mere absence of disease; optimal requirements are, in many circumstances, significantly greater. The large hang-up? Nutritionists as a group seem to be committed to holding the line and not giving an inch to the health food crowd. The quality of our diet has deteriorated progressively for decades, and every new survey shows it. It takes a big person to be the first to admit the situation is far from satisfactory. Vitamin E has always been a particularly hard nut to swallow. We 'fortify' (foods) with thiamine, riboflavin, niacin and iron. Why not vitamin E?"

"Most persons over this age may in fact be unwitting candidates without having any satisfactory way to identify it," says Dr. Barker. "Some suggest that accelerated aging may represent a sign of prolonged mild deficiency (of vitamin E). Our increasing incidence of degenerative diseases occurring in ever younger populations may represent another sign of it."

He goes on to remind us of the experiments of Dr. Lester Packer who was able to extend the life of human cells growing in a laboratory tissue culture from 50 generations to 116 generations just by adding extra vitamin E to the culture. "It is no myth that vitamin E is important in retarding aging of our cells."

"Vitamin E supplements are particularly important for an estimated 50 million world-wide users of the contraceptive pill, to minimize risk of venous thrombosis (blood clots). Those exposed to X-ray treatment for cancer therapy as well as those requiring prolonged oxygen therapy are also candidates for benefit from supplements of vitamin E," Dr. Barker continues.

Dr. Barker says we should think of nutrition as our best method of "rust-proofing" our bodies. But, he says, just getting the right kind of food at meals is not enough these days. First, the foods are depleted of nutrients by being transported long distances, then stored, then frozen and thawed, cooked and drained. We also use too much of drugs like aspirin and antibiotics, alcohol, diuretics (water pills), sugar, tobacco and tranquilizers, added to the stress of illness, surgery, injuries, domestic and work stress, all of which have been shown to increase our need for nutrients. "It is not surprising," he says, "that more and more people are discovering that they feel better when they supplement their diets regularly."

Dr. Barker warns, as have the Drs. Shute, against taking more than 200 units of vitamin E if you suffer from chronic rheumatic heart disease, severe heart failure or uncontrollably high blood pressure. It seems that getting very large doses of vitamin E may complicate these conditions.

A brilliant Canadian biochemist, David Turner, worked with NASA in solving the problem of anemia in astronauts. This came about because of lack of vitamin E caused by breathing pure oxygen for long periods of time. By the same token, Dr. Turner believes that ozone in air pollution may be creating the same kind of deficiency in our urban population. So this factor alone may have greatly increased our needs for vitamin E. (Recent reports have indicated possible ozone trouble for passengers on long transcontinental flights).

Dr. A. L. Tappel of the University of California has found that **protection against air pollution increases in direct proportion to the amount of vitamin E being taken**. Another researcher, Dr. D. N. DiLuzio, found, in 78 out of 81 persons tested, a high ratio of certain kinds of unhealthful fats which are formed in the absence of enough vitamin E to prevent peroxidation. These fats have been correlated with heart disease. Giving vitamin E reduced the amounts of such fats that could be found.

Dr. Max K. Horwitt, biochemist of St. Louis University, has conducted an eight-year study of human deficiency in vitamin E. He recently warned of the potential danger to people who are exposed to smog. Dr. Horwitt, who was one of the earliest researchers concerned with this vitamin, **believes that we should be getting from 200 to 800 units of the vitamin daily**, as we reported in Chapter I. Dr. Horwitt adds that it is impossible to design any experiments that will evaluate the full effects of prolonged vitamin E deficiency—that is, deficiency over 30 to 40 years.

The power of vitamin E is illustrated dramatically in another issue of *The Summary*. An Ontario physician, Dr. John K. MacKenzie, tells the remarkable story of **a patient with diabetes who came to the doctor complaining of severe impairment of vision**. Earlier he had experienced "whiteouts" of vision. An ophthalmologist had found elevated blood sugar and eye hemorrhages.

A thorough investigation at a hospital indicated that the impaired vision was due to diabetic retinopathy—a diseased retina due to diabetes. The patient had a family history of diabetes. He had smoked three packs of cigarettes a day for more than 30 years and had recently switched to a pipe. He had some symptoms of the vascular disease intermittent claudication in which there is severe pain when walking, due to obstruction of the blood vessels in the legs.

The hospital gave him a very gloomy prognosis. The impairment of his vision involved primary central vision.

42

The man was a commercial artist. He was about ready to give up his job and sell his car, since it was becoming impossible to work or to drive.

Says Dr. MacKenzie, "In my office while standing three feet from my medical diploma hanging on the wall, he was quite unable to read any of the script. He said he had the impression he had been medically abandoned."

Dr. MacKenzie placed him on 1,600 I.U. of vitamin E daily and later increased this to 2,000 units. He saw him frequently to check on his progress. And progress it surely was! Within a few weeks he was able to read uppercase print in the *Readers Digest*. His ability to exercise improved so greatly that he was able to walk greater distances with less pain. His blood sugar became much easier to control. (This is a usual occurrence with diabetics on vitamin E. Those on insulin must have frequent checks on blood sugar, since, with vitamin E in large doses, it may sink too low).

The diabetic patient bought another car and returned to his job as an artist, able to see well enough to continue his work and to drive. He returned to the ophthalmologist who had examined him several months before. According to Dr. MacKenzie, "The ophthalmologist, in reviewing his file for comparison, expressed astonishment at his recent findings, using the words 'dramatic' and 'miraculous.'"

Another patient, a 70-year-old fisherman in Halifax, N.S., had been severely diabetic for many years, taking very large doses of insulin daily. He was now suffering from extensive ulceration of the left foot with gangrenous changes including the toes. Because of the seriousness of his condition, Dr. MacKenzie suggested that he enter the hospital so that his blood sugar could be better controlled and his leg possibly amputated, if it could not be saved.

The old man refused. He didn't want to go to a Halifax hospital. Dr. MacKenzie asked if he would take vitamin E in large doses. He agreed to do so. Says Dr. MacKenzie, "The story had a happy ending. A man whose daily habit was to sit in the kitchen with his left leg supported on a kitchen chair became fully ambulatory and the ulcerative areas completely healed. The areas of blackish discoloration disappeared and a grossly swollen foot became the match of its counterpart."

Says Dr. MacKenzie, **"My experience over the years seems to indicate that the large body of vitamin E agnostics is shrinking.** As they should. For those cases which I considered had a reasonable chance to respond to vitamin E intake, one has never really had a failure yet. I also believe that in most cases, vitamin C should be taken concomitantly with vitamin E and that also in adequate doses.

"Vitamin E has travelled far from London, Ontario and the world literature is now heavily endowed with multiple references on vitamin E therapy. I admire the pioneers who have shown the way through much unnecessary and unwarrranted adversity, because it was only through their perseverance that vitamin E is becoming so well recognized as an established therapeutic agent."

In an earlier issue of *The Summary*, Dr. Evan Shute carried a full account of a symposium on vitamin E which was held in Hakone, Japan in September, 1970. Dr. Shute spoke at the conference on the history of vitamin E. Some excerpts follow.

Vitamin E was discovered in 1922. A Danish veterinarian used it in 1932 for "habitual abortion" in animals. At that time the only vitamin E available was wheat germ oil, with several International Units per dram, and a synthetic vitamin E tablet with 10 units. In 1939 there was a conference in London on this vitamin. No one had a very clear idea as to just what they should do with this new vitamin and most of the papers read then had to do with obstetrics.

In 1949, another conference was held in New York. Here the various scientists talked about using the vitamin for heart cases, for burns and scars. The suggested dosage for treatment had risen to 300 or 400 units daily. Dr. Shute notes that the situation seemed so discouraging that no one present at that conference is working with vitamin E today, except the Shute brothers and their colleagues.

In 1955, another conference was held in Venice. At this meeting participants talked of eye disease, heart and circulatory problems and diabetes, in relation to vitamin E. But, says Dr. Shute, no one present at that meeting is today working with the vitamin. They have all given up and turned to other fields of research.

In 1955, Dr. Shute presented at a meeting of the British Medical Association and the Canadian Medical Association an exhibit of colored pictures of Shute patients treated with vitamin E. He proposed that they be shown at the

Vitamin E Content of Some Common Foods

Food	Vitamin E in one serving mg.
Beef	0.63
Eggs, 2	2.00
Liver	1.62
Oatmeal	2.10
Haddock	1.20
Brown rice	2.40
Baked potato	0.05
Turnip greens	2.30
Baked beans	1.16
Fresh peas	1.73
Wholegrain bread, 4 slices	2.2
Margarine, 1 tbsp	2.60
Soya oil, ½ cup	120.00
Mayonnaise, 1 tbsp	3.16
Wheat germ, ½ cup	27.00

American Medical Association convention. "I told the people I talked to there that if I was right the American profession should be allowed to see what we had done. If we were wrong, the quickest way to destroy us was to put our work up before the medical profession and let it be criticized," says Dr. Shute.

His exhibit was rejected on the grounds that it was "embarrassing" and "there was no room for it." "I mentioned in reply that I had been in the Convention Hall in Atlantic City; after all the exhibits were set up, there would still be room for two freight trains there. The refusal held and was repeated the following year. We never again will try for an exhibit at an American Medical meeting," said Dr. Shute.

"I saw Hiroshima here in Japan," he goes on. "It moved me profoundly, especially when **I recalled that I had urged the use of vitamin E for the self-treatment of burns in 1939** and Hiroshima waited till 1945 to offer this treatment its ultimate test. The fact that vitamin E was not used, the fact that it would not be used if we had another Hiroshima in Cairo or Jerusalem tomorrow, point to a monstrous medical iniquity. It was once proposed to put vitamin E on the Quaker ship, *Phoenix*, which sailed to Viet Nam, but medical advice hindered such help.

". . . I should add," continues Dr. Shute, "that many vitamins beside vitamin E have had a hard time gaining acceptance, especially vitamin C, but also vitamin A and nicotinic acid (a B vitamin), for example. It is difficult for medical authorities, once they have taken a stand, to reverse themselves. Then, too, nutrition is on the very fringe of medicine. There are very few courses on the subject in medical schools. Another difficulty is that doctors are taught to cure but not to prevent disease, and nutrition is really a parameter of prevention. . . .

"**Looking back over this rather somber history, one is impressed by the versatility of vitamin E**, the fundamental role it plays which makes it so helpful in so many

46

pathological conditions, and the state of medical mind in our day which still believes only what Galen said and refuses to make the simplest therapeutic trial, for instance on burns. This story will appear unbelievable to our successors 20 years away. But meantime, imagine the sum of pain and disability for which the same medical incredulity that rejected vitamin C for nigh on two centuries has been responsible here."

This brings us to the best food sources of vitamin E. Think of them in relation to the amount of each that you might eat in the course of a day. You eat liver and oatmeal in average servings. You eat a serving of peas or baked beans, brown rice, turnip or other greens at a meal. All these contain ample vitamin E. Although soybean oil along with other salad oils, is very rich in vitamin E, you cannot get down "a serving" of soybean oil at one meal, and you shouldn't. Salad oils are highly concentrated foods. But you can and should use them in smaller quantities wherever appropriate—in salads, for instance, and recipes where you might otherwise use butter or hydrogenated shortening.

As might be expected, wholegrains contain more vitamin E than white flour or processed cereals, since most of the vitamin E in grains is concentrated in the germ and bran which are removed during processing. Adding insult to injury, bleaching of flour to make it chalky white destroys the last of whatever vitamin E was in the white flour or processed cereal to begin with. The two parts of the grain which are removed, the germ and the bran, are rich sources of vitamin E.

A serving of wheat germ (3½ ounces) contains 27 units of vitamin E. All whole, unrefined seeds contain it, as well as green leafy vegetables and eggs. There are, of course, many food supplements containing vitamin E.

CHAPTER 3

Vitamin E and Heart Disease

THE ROYAL COLLEGE OF PHYSICIANS in England recently issued a report on heart disease in which they blamed fatty foods such as meat, eggs and milk as the chief culprits in heart and circulatory conditions. Dr. T. L. Cleave, who has written a great deal on the subject of sugar and other refined carbohydrates in regard to heart disease, took them to task in the May 29, 1976 issue of the *British Medical Journal*.

Said Dr. Cleave with his customary logic and vigor, "The keeping of flocks of sheep, herds of cattle and other domestic animals in order to provide a continuity of meat and milk started with Neolithic man many thousands of years before the Christian era, and even only 1,400 years before that era Moses was stating that Jehovah gave to his people to eat 'butter of kine, and milk of sheep, with fat of lambs.' In a recent work I considerably amplified this, but to disregard any question of religion there remain the evolutionary implications.

"The first of these involves the time factor, based on history. The times of Moses were around 1400 B.C., when he led the Israelites away from the Pharoah of Egypt (probably Seti I or Rameses II). Contrast this date with the explosion of coronary thrombosis (heart attack) which dates from about 1920 in most Westernized countries like our own. If we allow for the 'incubation period' in coronary thrombosis, which may often amount to 30 years from the first impact of the cause, it would seem much more plausible to seek that cause in the enormous rise in sugar consumption, which, as I pointed out in 1956, rose from some 15 pounds per head per year in 1815 to the very high level of some 100 pounds per head per year around 1890 and over 120 pounds per head per year today. As opposed to this 800% rise, fat consumption has probably risen by only about 25 to 50%.

"The second implication concerns the naturalness, or the lack of it, of any foods discussed. The consumption of animal fats has been natural to man, as I have said, since far more remote times than those of Moses, times when man was primarily a hunter."

Dr. Cleave goes on to point out that during all those years of hunting and gathering (as the archeologists call it), human beings had very little access to any vegetable oils like our present salad oils. Early man had no mechanical equipment for making oils from any kind of seeds. Hence, says Dr. Cleave, salad oils (now being much praised as being more desirable than butter, fatty meat or cream) are really not a "natural" food for human beings at all, so how can experts decide that they are preferable to butter and other fats of animal origin, in preventing heart and circulatory conditions?

"Readers of this report," he said, "cannot be blamed if they deeply ponder these points before deciding, often against their instinct of taste, to fight shy of such ancient foods, often held in such high medical esteem, as milk, butter, and the 'fat of lambs.'"

In the same issue of the *British Medical Journal*, a British scientist wrote also criticizing the report. Said Walter Yellowlees, "In East Africa the Masai and Sambura tribes eat enormous quantities of animal fat, amounting to

49

60% of their calories. But they do not suffer from coronary heart disease (CHD). In southeast England more butter, meat and total fats are consumed per head of population than in Scotland, but the Scots have a far higher death rate from CHD than do the inhabitants of Southeast England. The Victorian middle and upper classes were prodigious eaters of animal fats—but among them CHD was very rare. The scale of the increase in CHD during this century cannot be related to a similar increase in the consumption of fat. In America a 12% increase in fat consumption between 1909 and 1961 was due mostly to an increase in the supply of oils and unsaturated fats; during the same period there was a high increase in the death rate from CHD.

"Is, therefore, the dietary advice on the prevention of CHD given by the learned authors of the Joint Working Party report a lot of nonsense? When we learn of the full implications of that advice our suspicions of nonsense are confirmed. We must eat only three eggs weekly and a special brand of margarine instead of butter, while glorious cream is forbidden; in preparing scrambled eggs, our wives must discard the yolks and use coloring matter instead. But worse is to follow from enthusiasts of the fat theory. In Australia some unfortunate cows are being fed grains treated with formaldehyde-casein in order to interfere with digestive bacterial action and so prevent hydrogenation of unsaturated fats. All this in aid of a theory of the action of polyunsaturated fatty acids which has never been proved and which a DHSS panel recently repudiated.

"Until our cardiologists can give us evidence more convincing than a confused tangle of biochemistry, I shall continue to have my egg for my breakfast and my glass of milk at lunchtime and shall still believe in the truth of the old Scots adage, "Butter betters a 'thing'"

Robert J. Samuelson, writing in the *Washington Post*, traces the history of the decline in egg consumption in the United States. From 1945, long before the scare about cholesterol began, sales of eggs had dropped until annual

50

consumption per capita was only 314 rather than the 403 level of 1945. The egg producers claim—and we think justly—that advertising for processed breakfast cereals was the reason for the decline, along with a nationwide trend to pay far less attention to breakfast, get it over with in a hurry. That generally means just pouring some snap-crackle-pop goodies out of a box rather than bothering to prepare a nourishing breakfast. The processed cereal industry has doubled their sales in the years since 1948.

Egg producers, and a great many nutrition experts as well, say that comparing the nutritional value of processed cereals to eggs is like comparing rhinestones to diamonds. By 1971, however, insistence on the threat of cholesterol in eggs had worked its harm and the egg industry was in terrible condition. They began to advertise that there is no scientific evidence that eating eggs in any way increases the risk of heart attacks. The American Heart Association got upset and went to the Federal Trade Commission. The FTC decided that, on the basis of the theories of a number of prominent scientists, it was untruthful to advertise like this and told the egg industry to stop.

Meanwhile, the cereal industry is spending about $80 million annually to advertise their sugar-laden products, whose nutritional worth is recognized as practically nil by almost every scientist except those working directly or indirectly for the cereal industry. So far the FTC has looked the other way, even though many consumer groups have done powerful work in presenting evidence against processed cereals before congressional committees in Washington.

What's the story on eggs? Is there any reliable evidence that they increase the risk of heart attacks? Not so far as we are concerned. They contain the finest protein available. Egg protein serves as the standard against which all other proteins are measured. Eggs contain all the vitamins in good quantity except vitamin C and all minerals we need. They are especially desirable for their fine iron content and

51

their sulfur. They contain more cholesterol than any other food except perhaps liver and kidney, which are the two other wholly natural foods richest in all nutrients except starch. Nutrition experts who work for the cereal industry also counsel against eating either of these two fine foods.

Why? Human beings have been eating them for millions of years. Along with eggs they have been the protein mainstay of nutritious diets for all the years of history and pre-history. **Heart attacks as such were never diagnosed or found at autopsy until early in this century**. How could eggs and other protein foods rich in cholesterol be the villains?

Highly processed breakfast cereals have been available for only the past few years. Sugar—and many of the new cereals are more than half sugar—has never been available for the general public except in teaspoons (like a spice) until early in this century. How can anybody doubt that sugar and other refined carbohydrates, not fat and certainly not cholesterol, are responsible for our heart and artery problems?

We turned up a new bit of evidence against processed cereals in a recent issue of the *American Journal of Clinical Nutrition*. Two scientists at the University of Georgia fed laboratory rats on processed cereals in different combinations, some sugary, some just starchy, some with considerable protein content. The animals suffered from many kinds of disorders and early death. They had high blood pressure, high cholesterol levels, fatty livers, anemia, unhealthful collections of iron in the liver and much more. There was no animal fat in any of these diets. No cholesterol. How then did it happen that cholesterol levels in the blood soared in some animals? In other animals blood cholesterol was low and in every case where this was so, the liver of the animal was fatty. The cholesterol was collecting in the liver rather than in the blood.

Compare this with an experiment performed by that master of nutritional good sense, Dr. Roger J. Williams of the University of Texas, who fed a group of rats on nothing at all but eggs for their entire lifetimes. They lived in perfect health far longer than most such animals live and far longer than the control rats, all of which got diets consisting of only one food: either milk, or hamburger, frankfurters, canned tuna, roasted peanuts, enriched wheat flakes or enriched puffed rice. We have listed these in terms of their contribution to good health and growth. Rats eating the enriched commercial cereals weighed less and were in poorer health at the end of 100 days than at the beginning of the experiment. Twenty-nine animals died of malnutrition on their inadequate diets. No rats eating the all-egg diet died. How can anyone believe that such a fine food as the egg can bring ill health?

This brings us to a discussion about a substance which may very well protect you against heart disease—vitamin E. In 1974, *Prevention* magazine asked their readers to answer a questionnaire on vitamin E and its effects on their health. They received 20,000 replies, a magnificent testimony to the loyalty of health seekers who take vitamin E regularly and are willing to take the time and trouble to tell others about their experience.

The survey was conducted and studied by Richard A. Passwater, Ph.D., a biochemist, who has since written two very fine books on vitamin therapy, the first being *Supernutrition: The Megavitamin Revolution*; the second one, *Supernutrition for Healthy Hearts*. Dr. Passwater states in *Prevention* that a critical level which appears to influence the possibility of developing heart disease is 300 International Units of vitamin E daily. Occasionally, he says, "people taking 200 I.U. of vitamin E daily developed heart disease (generally in the late 80's) or showed little improvement. When they increased their dosage, they experienced improvement. Only one case of heart trouble was reported to have developed at a higher dosage level." This was in the group of people responding to the survey who were 80 years old or older.

"The suggestion emerges," says Dr. Passwater, **"that**

among persons over 80, taking 1,200 I.U. or more of vitamin E daily after a heart attack improves chances of complete recovery and that taking 300 I.U. or more of vitamin E daily for 10 years or longer reduces the chances of ever developing heart disease. There is also a hint (in the replies that came in) that eating a balanced diet even in absence of vitamin E supplements has a considerable protective effect against heart disease. This survey supports those observations but does not prove them."

In the following issues of *Prevention*, Dr. Passwater reviewed comments from people of the various age groups who replied to the survey. Testimony was almost unbelievable—of heart trouble overcome, circulatory symptoms overcome, much more vigor and freedom from pain, as well as many comments on conditions other than circulatory ones, comments which were volunteered by the respondents although they had not been asked to say anything on these ailments.

The 50- to 59-year-old age group consisted of replies from 6,205 men and women. Of these 818 had heart disease. Correlating the replies, Dr. Passwater found that:

1. Taking 400 I.U. or more of vitamin E is strongly associated with reducing the incidence of heart disease to one-tenth or less of the risk for this age group in a general population not taking the vitamin.

2. Taking 1,200 I.U. or more of vitamin E for four years or more is strongly associated with reducing the risk of heart disease to less than one-third of the risk for this age group in the general population.

3. More than 80 per cent of the people who responded to the survey who already have heart conditions (including tachycardia, angina and fibrillation) reported that their condition improved when they used vitamin E.

Here are some striking comments from people in this age group. A woman had two heart attacks 15 years ago, has taken 400 units of vitamin E ever since. No more attacks. Another woman had fibrillation (rapid disorganized heartbeat) and high blood pressure. She has been taking 800 I.U. for 10 years, has had no more attacks and now has a natural heart rhythm. A husband with a heart attack is now taking 1,200 units of vitamin E; his wife, also victim of a heart attack, takes 800 units daily. The vitamin has lowered their blood pressure and their cholesterol count and "helped both hearts to heal." A woman whose heartbeat was 200 per minute put herself on 800 units of vitamin E when the doctors could do nothing for her. She has been well since.

Of the group of people 60 to 69 years of age who responded to the survey, Dr. Passwater says, "Perhaps the single most important age group to study for heart disease is the 60 to 69 year old group. This age group has a high incidence of heart disease and still includes in its numbers those individuals who are destined not to survive beyond the average life span." They had 6,459 replies to the questionnaire, of whom 1,543 said they have heart disease. Their replies showed, in general, what the younger group had shown—that 400 units of vitamin E daily for 10 years or more reduces the incidence of heart disease to one-tenth or less of the risk for people not taking the vitamin. Taking 1,200 units or more for four years or more seems to reduce the risk of heart disease to less than one-third of the risk for this age group. More than 80 per cent of those with heart trouble reported the vitamin improved their condition.

Says Dr. Passwater, **"You can't take vitamin E as a preventive measure and do everything else wrong**. If you smoke, drink, are inactive, overstrain, don't rest or eat properly, taking a pound of vitamin E daily won't completely protect you from heart disease, especially if you are genetically prone to it. However, you could be better off than if you didn't take any vitamin E at all."

Some comments from the respondents in their 60's are illuminating. A woman reported on curing her angina and heart murmur with 400 units of vitamin E. When she stopped taking the vitamin for six months, both these conditions returned. She began again and her problems vanished. A woman with coronary thrombosis and phlebitis reported that both improved greatly when she took vitamin E. A man with three coronary attacks and hardening of the arteries reported that he gave up his nitroglycerin tablets one year after starting vitamin E—800 units daily. Another man testified that a number of friends who are also M.D.'s have had coronaries and are all taking from 800 to 1,200 units of vitamin E daily. A man with severe pains from angina increased his intake of vitamin E from 100 to 400 units daily with a slight improvement. When he increased it to 800 units, "the improvement was fantastic," he says.

From the group of *Prevention* readers who are in their 70's, 4,060 replies were received. The same trend appears in this group: people who have taken 300 or more units of vitamin E daily for 10 years or more are not likely to develop heart disease. And neither are people taking 1,200 units or more daily for more than three years.

Many of the people in their 70's wrote of pain treated with vitamin E. A 75-year-old man said, "I would awaken every morning early about 4 or 5 a.m. with my eyeballs hurting, severe pains in the temples and back of the neck. I was also nauseated. I felt like I was losing my mind. In just two weeks of 800 units of vitamin E the condition improved and has been relieved ever since."

A 74-year-old man with a coronary 30 years ago has been taking 1,200 units of vitamin E daily and has had no recurrence. A 75-year-old woman had angina pectoris and weakness of heart valves. She has been taking vitamin E for 22 years, is at present taking 2,400 units daily. Her blood pressure has dropped to a healthy 120/80; her cholesterol level is down to 150.

A 71-year-old woman has been taking vitamin E since 1958, after a Mayo Clinic diagnosis of such severe heart damage that she required surgery. She has been taking high doses of vitamin E since 1958, is now taking 600 units daily.

Her doctors say she has no heart damage and very little angina pain.

A 71-year-old woman had been taking two heart medications plus three kinds of diuretics and had been told by her doctors that she could not ever live without digitalis. She started taking 1,000 units of vitamin E daily. By gradually increasing her vitamin and mineral intake, she is now able to do without any drugs. She now takes 800 units of vitamin E.

Dr. Passwater says, in part, ". . . these comments are not accepted as scientific proof that vitamin E prevents or cures heart disease. Rigid controlled studies involving 'double-blind' tests are required for evidence of validity by most scientists. Yet the information is useful. I do not know of any large-scale, well-controlled, double-blind test that proves aspirin cures headaches. But physicians and lay people 'know' it does through experience.

"Similarly many physicians know that vitamin E relieves angina pain and prescribe it; others have tried it and not seen the improvement described here, and still other physicians refuse even to try vitamin E. The main obstacle seems to be that many physicians have not considered the dose-time relationship required. They have tried too-little dosage for a too-little time. Now they should test the 300-plus units for 10-plus years, or 1,200-plus units for three-plus years."

What about people in their 80's who answered the questionnaire? Here are some comments from them. In this group the same general conditions prevailed—the level of 300 units of vitamin E daily appeared to influence the risk of heart disease. Dr. Passwater believes the figures he collected show that in those over 80, taking 1,200 units of vitamin E daily after a heart attack improves chances of complete recovery and taking 300 units daily for 10 years or more reduces the chances of having a heart attack.

One 84-year-old woman has been taking vitamin E for 30 years. She has been experimenting with dosage and with other elements in diet and way of life. She is now taking 500 to 600 units of vitamin E and is in excellent health. An 86-year-old man had two heart attacks years ago, began taking 1,800 units of vitamin E daily and has now been free of heart attacks for 25 years. An 81-year-old woman with phlebitis and a leg ulcer has been taking vitamin E for 25 years, mostly in doses of 1,000 units daily. All her circulatory problems have cleared up. Another 81-year-old woman had a coronary thrombosis (heart attack caused by a blood clot) 20 years ago. Fifteen years ago she began to take vitamin E and is now in very good health. An 86-year-old man has no more angina pains since he began to take 600 units of vitamin E daily for six years.

Many other fascinating bits of testimony turned up in the *Prevention* survey. Although no questions were asked about conditions other than circulatory ones, a great deal of evidence came in on improvement in other conditions as well. And, most astonishing of all, 70 physicians answered the questionnaire, 66 of whom had been taking vitamin E from one to 29 years. An 89-year-old physician (and isn't that some kind of a record?) treats himself and his patients with vitamin E. He had very serious heart trouble 26 years ago. He has taken 800 units of vitamin E daily for 26 years. A man described as a "well known" New York physician reported to *Prevention* that his last electrocardiogram and blood pressure are normal after two years of taking 1,000 units of vitamin E daily after a coronary thrombosis. Another doctor claims he cured his prostatitis with 800 units of vitamin E daily. That's the first such testimony we have read on that condition.

It is cheering indeed to read such valuable and unsolicited remarks from people who had suffered for years from one or another disease. And not one word of any unpleasant side effects from really immense doses of vitamin E. One can only wonder why official medicine does not realize the significance of all this and take another look at the harm they may be doing with pills and surgery, when the answer for most people may lie in a small capsule of a perfectly natural substance taken regularly every day for life.

In the *Proceedings of the Canadian Federation of Biologists Society*, Vol. 14:45, 1971, two scientists reported on changes in the hearts of rats made deficient in vitamin E. The rats were kept on a vitamin E deficient diet for 10 weeks. Their hearts showed a number of alterations from normal in the process of energy production.

And in the *Canadian Journal of Physiology and Pharmacology*, Vol. 49: 909, 1971, three scientists also found decided changes in the heart and heart function in animals made deficient in vitamin E. They also found that it was necessary to feed the animals plenty of vitamin E for longer than four weeks for complete recovery from some of these symptoms.

In a letter to *Canadian Family Physician*, Vol. 19, page 15, 1973, a Canadian physician, **Dr. M. Lattey, reports on his personal experience taking vitamin E for paroxysmal auricular fibrillation.** This is extremely rapid, irregular and dangerous heart contractions. The doctor began with 400 units of vitamin E, which proved to be not enough. He doubled it, taking 800 milligrams of vitamin E daily and his heart returned to normal.

He reported that he now is able to exercise without any difficulty and says he has not enjoyed such good health for seven years. He adds that the medical profession should take another look at the use of vitamin E for heart disease.

In a Polish medical journal, *Fortschiritte du Med.*, Vol. 90, Supplement 913, 1972, a Polish physician reports on 29 patients with many of the heart and artery symptoms which are becoming commonplace among people who live in Western industrialized societies. These patients ranged in age from 38 to 72 years.

Fifteen were suffering from coronary and circulatory problems, plus angina pectoris, myocardial infarct, claudication, fatty liver and high blood levels of fats.

Ten patients had high levels of cholesterol, fatty livers, diabetes and circulatory troubles. Four patients had fatty livers, high levels of cholesterol, obesity and badly functioning thyroid glands.

All were given six capsules of vitamin E, with 150 milligrams in each capsule. As their condition improved, this dosage was reduced by half. In all cases, the level of blood fats went down within a few weeks. In some cases, cholesterol levels were lowered by 100 per cent or more. In other cases blood fats were lowered by 36 per cent, angina pains decreased and claudication improved. This is a painful disorder which occurs in patients when they try to walk, with leg arteries blocked with fatty deposits. Diastolic blood pressure fell an average of 15 mm of mercury. There were no harmful side effects.

Purpura means hemorrhages in the skin, mucus membranes and other parts of the body. An article from the *Journal of Vitaminology* (published in Japan), Vol. 18, page 125, 1972, tells of seven cases of purpura treated with vitamin E. **Four hundred to 600 milligrams of the vitamin were given daily and there was "marked clinical improvement."** Six out of the seven cases improved with vitamin E therapy alone.

It is interesting to note that, **at the same time, the vitamin improved other conditions as well**, such as local swelling (or edema) and skin eruptions. The authors believe this demonstrates that vitamin E prevents damage to capillary walls when this damage is due to drugs, infections and so on.

An Italian physician reported in *Gynecol. Practique*, Vol. 22, page 501, 1971, that **he treated with vitamin E 48 women complaining of menopausal troubles**. He believes, he says, that vitamin E has many beneficial effects, even on the genital organs. It protects the nervous system and muscles, and deters hardening of the arteries. It "tunes the metabolism" of carbohydrates. In Italy vitamin E is widely used in treating aging, he says, and especially hardening of the arteries. Eighty-one per cent of the women he treated with vitamin E were helped through a difficult menopause.

A letter to the editor of *The American Journal of Clinical Nutrition*, Vol. 26, page 382, 1973, tells of the writer's fears that large doses of vitamin E may affect the liver adversely as well as the levels of vitamin C and vitamin A. He says that, in rats, only small doses are safe. Could the same be true of human beings?

Dr. Evan Shute, who edits *The Summary* and who is one of the world's leading authorities on vitamin E, comments as follows: "I have taken 800 to 1,600 I.U. of vitamin E daily for 40 years and my liver still works well. Others have taken 400 to 8,000 units daily for many years—always with safety. Thousands of *humans* (not rats) we know have used 400 to 1,600 I.U. daily for years with never any indication of either liver problems ensuing or vitamin A toxicity. We know—we don't need to extrapolate scientific (?) guestimates. This illustrates once again that rats are not men. Biochemists must remember this."

In a recent issue of the *New England Journal of Medicine*, a British Columbia physician reported on the **use of vitamin E for relief of angina pectoris**. This is the severe chest pain which accompanies certain heart conditions. Says Dr. W. M. Toone, he treated 22 men from 61 to 73 years old. He gave 11 of them a capsule containing nothing and the other 11 received capsules of vitamin E (400 units four times daily).

In addition to the vitamin treatment, he had already instituted a therapeutic program for these patients in which they gave up smoking, took long walks every day, lost weight, ate meals with low cholesterol and triglyceride content (these are fatty substances) and avoided stress of all kinds. Now keep in mind that all the patients were on this therapy program—not just the ones getting vitamin E.

The doctor studied the 22 men for two years. During this time three patients in each group reduced considerably the amount of nitroglycerin they had to take to relieve the angina pain. In addition, four patients who were getting the vitamin E reduced their nitroglycerin to one or two tablets a month—that is, almost none. No one in the group getting the "dummy" capsule was able to do this. So it appears, says the doctor, that the vitamin E capsules brought such improvement that the patients taking them could eliminate almost entirely the nitroglycerin pain pill which they had been taking regularly.

"We have had no complications after the use of vitamin E; although it is a fat-soluble vitamin, there have been no cases of toxicity that we have noted even with the very high doses used. A recent report of muscular weakness by H. M. Cohen has not been duplicated in any of our cases. On the contrary, there has been a sense of well-being in taking vitamin E."

Dr. Toone was referring here to a *California Medicine* article by a California physician whose letter to the *New England Journal of Medicine* follows his own. Dr. H. M. Cohen tells what seems to us an incredible story. He decided, he says, to put some of his patients on vitamin E. He gave them 800 milligrams daily and decided to take the same amount himself. His partner also said he would volunteer to take 800 milligrams of vitamin E daily.

Things went uneventfully until one week later when, Dr. Cohen says, he began to feel terribly weak and fatigued, "as if I were suffering from a severe influenzal syndrome." He stopped taking vitamin E and the weakness and fatigue disappeared. He said nothing of this to anyone, but started to take vitamin E again and found the same thing happening. His partner then revealed to him that he had been feeling very weak and fatigued. He stopped taking vitamin E and the trouble disappeared.

From then on, says Dr. Cohen, patients began calling to report that they, too, suffered from great weakness when they took vitamin E, which stopped when they discontinued it. Dr. Cohen says he has now investigated many people—especially young people—who come to him complaining of fatigue. Invariably, he says, they have been taking vitamin E and, as soon as they stop, their fatigue disappears.

In our numerous books and magazine articles, we have reported literally hundreds of cases of people taking this much or more vitamin E who have experienced nothing but feelings of great well-being, along with the diminishing of various complaints, mostly having to do with circulation, skin health and general fitness. Why or how, out of all the doctors who recommended vitamin E, only this one doctor and his partner should have this experience is beyond belief. Dr. Robert Atkins, of New York, for example, who treats overweight and obese patients with a diet very high in protein and fat, with almost no carbohydrate, also gives vitamin E to all his patients—and he has case records of 11,000. They are told to take 800 units of vitamin E daily. He tells us that his patients report feelings of great well-being. They tell him they never felt so well as they feel on his prescribed diet and supplements.

A German veterinarian reports in a 1960 issue of *Tierarztliche Umschau* that he uses vitamin E for treating animals with heart conditions. A one-year-old poodle with heart trouble regained complete health after 14 days on vitamin E. A three-year-old thoroughbred horse with acute heart failure was treated with vitamin E for two weeks, after which time its electrocardiogram showed only trivial changes even after exercise. The vet uses, he says, very large doses of the vitamin.

Working with laboratory rats, Dr. L. H. Chen and two associates found that animals who were getting little vitamin E had much higher blood levels of cholesterol than those which had plenty of the vitamin. And when vitamin E was added to the former diets, the cholesterol levels promptly dropped. Another aspect of the diet was studied. Animals which were getting low-protein diets had higher cholesterol levels than those on high-protein diets.

Say the authors, writing in the June, 1972 issue of *The*

Journal of Nutrition, "The interrelationship of dietary protein and vitamin E level in altering serum cholesterol was apparent."

In *Physiology, Chemistry and Physics*, Vol. 5, page 319, 1973, **three researchers tell us that vitamins A, D, E and K—but especially vitamin E—are inhibitors of cholesterol**. That is, they help to control levels of this fatty substance in the blood and muscles. When rabbits are given a diet deficient in vitamin E, cholesterol rises in their blood. Giving vitamin E brings the level down. Other researchers have found that rats, chicks, calves and guinea pigs with muscular dystrophy have higher levels of cholesterol in their muscles than healthy animals. Higher levels of cholesterol have been reported, too, in human beings with muscular dystrophy. Scientists have reported that vitamin E participates in controlling cholesterol manufacture in the liver.

What can you do to prevent heart disease? This is one of a series of questions and answers found in a most informative booklet, *Common Questions on Vitamin E and Their Answers*, by the Medical Staff of the Shute Institute for Clinical and Laboratory Medicine, London, Canada.

The Shute Institute takes up first congenital heart disease—that is, heart disease with which one is born. They tell us it may be preventable by giving vitamin E to the father of the child before conception. In other words, the father should be taking vitamin E before he and his wife begin to think about having children. There is now good evidence that if the husband's sperm cells are activated by vitamin E, the child born from such a father is more apt to be perfectly formed—so that he will not have any defects which can be classified as "congenital heart disease."

"Rheumatic heart disease" is defined by the Shute doctors as a condition resulting from infection by a certain strain of strep germ. This is likely to occur after tonsilitis or serious colds. Antibiotics given to control the infection should do much to prevent rheumatic infection of the heart. But the patient's resistance and general good health are also extremely important and here is where vitamin E enters the picture.

Vitamin E helps to prevent scarring of the heart muscle and the heart valves. It strengthens flabby heart muscles, provides better oxygenation of tissues and restores the health of the interior walls of capillaries, which are the smallest of the blood vessels. The Shute doctors believe that it should be taken for years after the acute attack of rheumatic heart trouble, because the condition might recur even as long as five or 10 years after the initial illness.

"Hypertensive and arteriosclerotic heart disease" are those conditions which are called degenerative diseases. They are usually associated with high blood pressure. It is helpful to keep blood pressure normal, keep one's own nervous tension controlled and keep one's weight normal. The susceptibility to this condition seems to run in families. So people whose relatives have suffered from these conditions should be especially careful. Other conditions which also run in families and also tend to make one susceptible to this kind of heart condition are diabetes, underactive thyroid and conditions which involve high blood levels of cholesterol.

Say the Shute physicians, "Much has been written on the pros and cons of cholesterol in these heart diseases and especially coronary heart disease, but medical men are still very unsure of their ground here. Perhaps there is more to be gained by avoiding obesity and undue mental stress, reducing animal fats in the diet and maintaining physical activity than by paying attention to cholesterol." The Shutes tend to agree with another theory on what thickens artery walls. This theory states that small blood clots build up on the linings of arteries and eventually thicken them, with cholesterol complicating the picture only after this has occurred.

"Coronary Heart Disease is one of the major health

problems of our times. Sudden blood clots that cause sudden deaths from this disorder have been diagnosed only since 1912. Yet this condition is now the commonest killer of all diseases.

"**Probably it is of dietary origin,**" say the Shute physicians, "but the evidence for this is indirect and vague. Its rise corresponds with a method of milling wheat which rejects most of all of the germ, but also with the rise of the cigarette habit and the increase in motor exhaust gases. Perhaps all of these play a causative role." It is true that the condition can be much better treated than prevented. But many cases never can be treated, since the victim dies in the first attack.

The value of vitamin E in this condition is stressed by the Shute doctors, for it is a natural anticoagulant. That is, it keeps blood from forming unwanted clots in blood vessels. Then, too, it helps the body to build detouring blood vessels around spots where arteries are blocked by the "hardening" process. It keeps the walls of blood vessels healthy. It dissolves blood clots already formed.

Vitamin E may prevent or dissolve microscopic "sludging" in the tiniest of the blood vessels. "Sludge" here means exactly what it means in terms of sewage sludge—deposits of unwanted material floating around the blood. **Vitamin E improves oxygenation**—that is, the tissues can take up more oxygen when enough vitamin E is present. So these tissues can have more resistance, for oxygen is vital for this.

They have evidence, say the Shute physicians, that **vitamin E given in proper dosage, prolongs the life of those who have had coronary attacks and so should always be considered by those who want to prevent such attacks.**

"In general," this helpful little book continues, "one should advise patients who want to avoid heart attacks to be active and not sluggish, to maintain normal weight and avoid becoming fat, to take alpha tocopherol (vitamin E) daily in large doses, even from babyhood, and to learn to live with the stresses of our day—to develop a calm philosophy, in other words."

Another more complete book by the Shute Medical Staff is *The Heart and Vitamin E*—40 chapters which "give real hope to those who suffer from diseases of the heart and blood vessels." The price is $3.00.

CHAPTER 4

Vitamin E
and Aging

THE STARTLING EVIDENCE came from human cells kept alive
in a laboratory culture. Under normal laboratory conditions, such cells might live for 50 generations of cell
division. But when a small amount of vitamin E was added,
the human cells in the testube continued to reproduce
beyond more than 120 divisions. Then the scientists
conducting the research discontinued the experiment.

Drs. Lester Packer and James R. Smith of the
University of California stated that the cells appeared to
show no signs of old age. They were still completely normal
and going on about the healthy business of dividing, just as
they had when the experiment began. Scientists generally
accept the theory that cells have a built-in lifespan
depending on the inheritance of the individual. You inherit
a set of cells which will see you through to a healthy old age,
other things being equal. Or, because of a long line of short-
lived, unhealthy ancestors, you may have inherited a
tendency to succumb to many diseases and die at an early
age.

But now it seems that the magic of vitamin E may have
proved this theory to be false. **Perhaps just getting enough
and more than enough vitamin E may enable the individual**

with a poor heritage to live much longer than expected.

The California scientists deny that their research demonstrates anything like this, of course. According to *The New York Times* for September 2, 1974, they stated that the most immediate benefits of this world-shaking discovery will be to benefit scientists. Now they can keep human cells alive long enough in a laboratory to investigate human genetics and develop ways to tinker with the genetics of human cells. Then, too, researchers can use such long-living cells to evaluate the effects of environmental stress, like pollutants, on cell life.

So, said they, this doesn't mean at all that taking vitamin E will prolong life or will turn the clock back for a 40-year-old and make him or her feel like 18. And why not? Well, said another California researcher who has done much work with vitamin E, everybody gets so much vitamin E in their food that the body has large stored reserves to draw upon, hence getting any more would be useless.

This is the kind of argument some scientists use when they are confronted with laboratory experiments which prove beyond a shadow of a doubt that some extraordinary vital substance exists in a given vitamin which performs almost magically on individual cells. Now consider for a moment that the human cell under the microscope which went right on behaving like a young, vital cell way past the time when it should have stopped dividing, apparently contained enough vitamin E to be a healthy cell. There was no indication that these cells were deficient in vitamin E. But when more vitamin E was added, the effects were entirely different from what happened to other cells being studied, which had not been given extra vitamin E. Is it not possible that whole human beings might expect this same effect, since the vitamin affects individual cells that way and since human bodies are nothing but collections of human cells?

The other specious argument is, of course, that all modern Americans get as much vitamin E as they need, so extra amounts bring no benefits. One examination of this fallacy was reported in *The American Journal of Clinical Nutrition* for July, 1965. Four scientists bought food to feed a family for eight days, stressing vitamin E-rich foods like margarine and salad oils. They planned highly nutritious meals with plenty of wholegrain cereals and breads, lots of eggs, meat and leafy vegetables. These meals were far more nourishing in every nutrient than the average American eats. And certainly they contained far more vitamin E than most of us get with every day's meals.

Yet when these researchers analyzed the foods they had bought, they found that the overall daily average of vitamin E in such meals was only about 7½ milligrams, one-half of the amount officially specified as a daily allowance at that time. Considering that almost nobody actually eats such highly nutritious diets containing so much vitamin E as this, there seems to be very good reason for fearing that many, many Americans are short on this essential vitamin.

There is actually no way of knowing how much any individual may need or get of any vitamin, because of the great differences in individual physiological make-up and ways of eating and living. So there is no way to tell how many Americans get, in their daily meals, less vitamin E than they need for good health. The reason for lack of vitamin E is, largely, that the germ has been removed from our processed cereals and the vitamin E along with it. What little vitamin E may remain in white flour is destroyed when that flour is bleached with chlorine.

Yet some authorities on vitamin E continue to say that we cannot be short on vitamin E because we are not suffering, nationally, from any disease of vitamin E deficiency. How do they know we are not? How do they know that the circulatory and heart conditions which kill more of us than any other disease are not caused directly or indirectly by lack of vitamin E, combined with some unnatural circumstance of modern life—air pollution, for example?

70

Dr. A. L. Tappel, Professor of Nutrition at the University of California at Davis, a long-time expert on vitamin E, told the *Times* that **vitamin E does indeed protect living cells against a kind of chemical known as oxidants**. These chemicals can damage cells. Some of them are present in urban air pollution chiefly because of car exhausts. Exposing laboratory animals to such pollution, in about the same concentration to which city dwellers are exposed, damages lungs. Giving vitamin E in quite large amounts to the animals protects them from such damage. It's just that simple.

Yet the same scientists who conducted these experiments continue to say, well, there is no reason for human beings to take vitamin E to protect themselves from air pollution. They all get enough vitamin E from their food. Weren't the laboratory animals getting enough vitamin E from their food, too? And didn't extra vitamin E protect them from damage? Why in the world should not we poor, tormented victims of modern technology be encouraged to use whatever harmless, inexpensive substance we can find to protect us, in some measure, from the pollution which we cannot escape?

Drs. Packer and Smith went on to make two of the most highly contradictory remarks we have ever heard from scientists. "Vitamin E won't extend life in humans," they said, "except in the possible case where humans are subjected to severe environmental pollution." (Aren't we all?) And then they went on to say, according to the *Times*, "Even if vitamin E can't turn a 40-year-old into a 14-year-old, it might prevent an early death, or brain disease, heart attacks or senility. Of course, we don't know these things at all, yet."

And the two scientists, who have presumably been told for years that we all get plenty of vitamin E in our food, are now taking 200 milligrams of vitamin E daily in capsules!

Those of us who take considerable amounts of vitamin E regularly, along with other vitamins and minerals, and notice immeasurable improvement in our health, are told by some scientists and physicians that we just imagine it and we'd get the same results taking pills that contain nothing at all. Yet when inert human cells, which certainly have no ability to imagine good health, demonstrate extraordinary vigor and longevity just because of a little dab of vitamin E added to their culture, then we are told, "oh, well, just because vitamin E brought such immense benefits to individual cells we can't say that it would bring similar benefits to that whole assembly of human cells that make up a human being!" Why not?

Fortunately, as long as we have a free press in this country, the health seeker can discover facts like these from the California laboratory. And he can make up his own mind as to whether he wants to buy some vitamin E and see for himself whether it will perform the same miracle for him that it performed for the human cells in that laboratory.

Vitamin E for removing wrinkles, frown lines and crow's feet? That's what a letter to the editor of *New Scientist* claims (March 6, 1975). Jan Harris states that "there is considerable weight of scientific opinion to support the fact that vitamin E assists in acceleration of healing and preventing the formation of scar tissue when taken orally or when applied to a wound. It has been recommended for topical application to burns to promote healing and to prevent formation of scar tissue.

"The effect of vitamin application to the skin of the face has been studied by Dr. Hans Selye (University of Montreal) who found that it arrested the development of 'crow's feet,' frown lines and laughter lines . . . there appears to be a good case for advocating the supplementing of diet with extra vitamin E and for its application topically for rejuvenating the skin cells.

"Considerable work on this subject has been carried out by Wilfrid Shute of the Shute Institute, London, Ontario, Canada, which supports this view and this subject was dealt with by him at the international symposium of vitamin E held at University College, London, in September, 1974, where considerable persuasive evidence was addressed."

This is one of the most recent in a series of reports on the power of vitamin E to ameliorate the rate and/or effects of aging. We have been told that individual cells exposed to vitamin E divide healthfully many more times than cells with no extra vitamin E, which seems to indicate that the vitamin has some extraordinary power to prevent some of the ravages of old age.

Now it appears that we may be able to achieve some of these effects by applying the vitamin directly to the skin. Dr. Hans Selye is a noted researcher whose work has been mostly concerned with stress and its effects on living organisms.

A Louisiana State University professor believes he may have found **a key for preventing the aging process— vitamin E**. Dr. William A. Pryor, a chemistry professor, says in an article in *Scientific American*, August, 1970, that the effects of diets deficient in vitamin E are very similar to effects of radiation damage and aging. In all three instances there is structural damage to the membranes of cells.

Researchers studying cells have found in them some very unstable compounds they call "free radicals" which play an important part in many processes involving oxygen. These substances are involved in some kinds of cancer; radiation damage to cells occurs partly through the action of these rather mysterious substances. Free radicals are formed in the body during the process of oxidizing food and making it into energy. This process is very carefully regulated in the cell by enzymes which control the burning of fats. When free radicals are present, the process is stopped. The oxygen will not react with the enzymes to consume the fat.

But when enough vitamin E is present, the free radicals are restrained and the process goes on in a normal fashion. So the vitamin E protects from harm. If it is not present, the fatty substances collect into a dark brown debris which is called "age pigment." Now it appears they may have nothing to do with aging. Perhaps they are just symptoms of vitamin E deficiency. Dr. Pryor does not mention it, but doesn't it seem possible, too, that vitamin E may also be able to help protect the cell against the ravages of radiation?

Kraurosis and other senile vulvular states are troublesome senile conditions associated with itching. They are very common and are often poorly handled by estrogens (female sex hormones), the usual medication, reported *The Summary* in December, 1972. But vitamin E is very valuable for shrinking tender vaginas due to aging, senile leucorrhea, vulvar pruritis, (itching) leukoplakia of the cervix (this is a pre-cancerous condition) and vulva, and dyspareunia in the elderly (painful or difficult intercourse). Vitamin E is also helpful in diabetic and anal pruritis (itching), *The Summary* reported.

The patterns of aging are always distinctive, reports Dr. Roger J. Williams at a conference on aging sponsored by the Huxley Institute for Biosocial Research, New York City. One person may have a deteriorated memory long before he needs a walking cane. Another may need the cane and yet retain a marvelous memory. One may become bald while retaining his sex urge; another retains his hair while losing his sex urge, says Dr. Williams.

The University of Texas biochemist goes on to say that every individual has a highly distinctive pattern of blood vessels, often more distinctive than fingerprints...and vastly more important.

He adds that, if the subject were explored in more detail, it would probably be found that people who retain their eyesight while aging have better circulation to the eyes and retina than those who have visual impairment. Those who have excellent circulation to the brain may age without showing loss of memory or mental acuity.

"Just as biochemical individuality enters into all phases of aging, each individual has a characteristic pattern of nutritional needs and this pattern may vary widely from that of others," Dr. Williams continues. "A dietary regimen that might delay aging in one person might accelerate it in another.

"Nutrition has been neglected for decades by the medical profession, and there is general ignorance and lack of exploration into the facts or factors involved. Our staple foods are often trashy and do not provide the nutritional essentials for adequate maintenance and repair of body cells and tissues."

Dr. Williams adds that self-selection of food plays a large role in all this. In respect to two commonly consumed energy-yielding chemicals, self-selection often works badly. These are sugar and alcohol, he says.

We often hear that our much longer lives testify to the benefits of modern technology, modern medicine and modern ways of life. Yet, according to gerontologist, Dr. Nathaniel C. Calloway of the University of Wisconsin, "U. S. Senators elected between 1789 and 1960, who ate fried apples, hominy and fat back for breakfast lived an average of 68½ years. When a comparable group of persons are considered, namely senators who ate a modern menu, elected between 1931 and 1966, it is found that their average age at death was 69 years. This means that all our glamorous developments, diets, flashing lights, records, discoveries and medical care have added only one-half year to the life of senators."

Since vitamin E is related to our use of oxygen, it is interesting to note that, on October 2, 1974, the Associated Press reported from Miami that doctors at the Miami Heart Institute have found they can treat senility temporarily with oxygen at high pressure—"hyperbaric oxygen." Working in 1971 with a group of 19 senile patients, doctors treated them in an oxygen chamber for four weeks and found improvement in their condition, especially those who were also taking a diuretic drug for kidney treatment.

A new study was begun involving 38 patients from 65 to 75 years old. Eighteen of them were placed in the hyperbaric oxygen chamber for 10 days and were given the drug. Another group of similar patients were given the oxygen treatment without the drug. And the rest were untreated. At the end of 10 days, a psychological test was given which revealed that the patients who got both the oxygen and the drug were in the best mental condition, while those who got the oxygen alone were next best. All of the patients tended to regress to their original state in the following 10 weeks. The improvement was temporary.

Doctors are optimistic but do not wish to raise hopes which may later be shattered. Nor are they equipped to deal with an avalanche of requests for information and treatment. Two Florida businessmen have bought several hyperbaric oxygen chambers and are giving treatments for $50 each with no drugs involved. We have no reports on the effects of these treatments.

Senility is a disease of older folks in which the mind sometimes appears to be blank. Senile people have difficulty remembering, especially remembering events of the present time, although their memory of past events may be clear. Their conversation tends to wander. They repeat themselves often without knowing it.

A Canadian psychiatrist, Dr. Abram Hoffer, believes that this kind of mind damage can be prevented by massive doses of the B vitamin niacin, along with other vitamins and the best possible diet. Dr. Hoffer said, "I have had some elderly people who were becoming senile, who, after being on a good level of niacin and other vitamins for one or two months, fully regained their normal mental activity.... And in my own practice, any time a patient comes to me in a pre-senile state, who follows this program faithfully, usually just about in every case, comes out pretty quickly.... It is my ambition to bring every man to such a state of good mental health that, until he dies... he will be in full possession of his faculties."

76

Dr. Hoffer, who has treated thousands of schizophrenic patients successfully with massive doses of niacin (vitamin B3) and vitamin C, takes a number of vitamin supplements himself, in an effort to prolong his own life and his good health, both mental and physical. He takes daily 4 grams of niacin (or niacinamide), 4 grams of vitamin C, 800 units of vitamin E, 250 milligrams of thiamine (vitamin B1), 250 milligrams of pyridoxine (vitamin B6), vitamin A and vitamin D, some calcium and iron and a mineral supplement. He firmly believes that senility is a state of chronic malnutrition.

Since oxygen and vitamin E are so closely related, could we not, do you suppose, get the effects of the hyperbaric oxygen chamber by simply taking enough vitamin E? In this way, those who are senile or pre-senile might not experience just temporary relief of symptoms. The relief could perhaps be permanent, so long as the vitamin E treatment continues.

Vitamin E has been shown to prevent "blow-outs" in human red blood cells, according to a Tacoma, Washington scientist who reported his findings to an American Chemical Society meeting.

Medical Tribune asked Dr. Jeffrey Bland if this means that people may take vitamin E and live longer, healthier lives. He answered, in their August 18, 1976 issue, by saying that he cannot promise such things definitely. But, he said, you should be able to avoid accelerated aging if you take the "right amount" of vitamin E. And studies are now in progress to determine what that "right amount" may be.

This is how he made his discovery. Exposing a red blood cell to any substance that oxidizes the cholesterol in the cell membrane weakens the membrane and there is a "blow-out," or a "budded cell." Vitamin E apparently slows this process. The process is enhanced by exposing the cell to oxygen, to the chemical pollutants in smog, to cigarette smoke, X-rays or the sun. These oxidizers change the cholesterol into cholesterol hydroperoxide which does the

77

damage to the cell membrane.

Dr. Bland and his associates gave 24 human volunteers 600 units of vitamin E and then took samples of their blood. A similar number of volunteers gave blood without taking the vitamin E. The cells of both groups were then exposed to light and oxygen for 16 hours. As expected, the cells from those volunteers who had no vitamin E showed a "totally budded" condition. That is, the cell membranes had been totally destroyed.

But the blood cells from those volunteers who took the vitamin E showed only "a small number" of budded cells. **This seems to indicate that the cell walls were almost completely protected from this kind of destruction by only 600 milligrams of vitamin E.** To someone exposed to cigarette smoke, air pollution or any of the other thousands of pollutants which oxidize cell membranes, it appears that just taking vitamin E alone might give an enormous amount of protection.

In a second experiment, Dr. Bland mixed some normal red blood samples with some vitamin E and exposed the mixture to light and oxygen. Once again, he tells us, "The cells resisted membrane destruction at the same rate ... as the cells taken from those donors on the augmented vitamin E diet."

Said Dr. Bland, "The vitamin is a biological antioxidant that sits in the fatty layer of the cell membrane" as protection against the effects of "cellular aging." **He then recommended that people exposed to smog and/or cigarette smoke take vitamin E as protection against these poisons.** Since it is almost impossible to escape these two prevalent toxins in modern life, it seems that he has just recommended, as we do, that everyone should take vitamin E in quite large amounts. We are surely not living in a pristine environment. Every breath of air we take contains pollutants. Most of us, whether we smoke or not, are exposed almost continually to cigarette smoke, since someone is smoking almost everywhere we go.

Dr. Bland seems to feel there is an upper limit to the amount of vitamin E that is needed to protect us. Not that any vitamin E over this amount would be harmful, just that it wouldn't give us the protection the "right amount" gives. Considering the vast amount of evidence that has appeared in medical and scientific journals, much of which we have discussed in this book, it seems to us that "the right amount" which can possibly be determined within the confines of a laboratory has little relevance to the vast majority of us human beings who deal with varying degrees and amounts of pollution and who smoke or do not smoke, and who are otherwise exposed or not exposed to the welter of chemicals that surround us every day.

In addition to this, there is the question of biological individuality. Each of us is born with a different need for vitamins and minerals and other nutrients. Some of us may need 20 or more times more of these than others. If someone whose needs have always been greater because of inherited tendencies happens to be the person whose exposure to pollutants is very great, surely such a person would need more of the vitamin than someone whose needs from birth are smaller and who somehow manages to escape many pollutants possibly by living in a remote area, avoiding tobacco smoke and so on.

Should you take 600 milligrams of vitamin E daily in the hope that it may help you to avoid damage from pollution and also early aging? We see no reason why you shouldn't. Should you hope, if you do, that you will live forever and will forever appear to be no older than 25? It doesn't seem likely that such a future can be achieved from taking any vitamin or from following any regimen of diet and supplements. We all age eventually.

But surely it is worthwhile to achieve whatever we can in the way of good health and postponement of disabled old age as long as we can. And it seems quite likely, from Dr. Bland's experiments and those of many other scientists that as much as 600 milligrams of the vitamin might provide that postponement. Along with a highly nutritious diet, plenty of rest and exercise.

Damage to chromosomes, the genetic material in cells, has been linked to cancer and the aging process, according to the May, 1973 issue of *Proceedings of the National Academy of Sciences*. If we could prevent the damage to chromosomes perhaps we could prevent cancer and retard aging.

Vitamin E, vitamin C and two other antioxidants have now been shown to reduce damage to chromosomes in blood cells exposed to chemicals known to be cancer-causing. Vitamin E gave 63.8 per cent protection against chromosome breakage, and vitamin C gave 31.7 per cent protection.

CHAPTER 5

Vitamin E and Air Pollution

IN THE September 28, 1974, *Science News* appears the information that two California scientists, Lester Packer and James R. Smith of the University of California, added vitamin E to human cells taken from very young tissues. Such cells as these would normally divide and reproduce about 50 times before dying. When the vitamin E was added, cells went right on dividing, in perfect good health, and had divided 120 times when the scientists wrote their articles on the subject. *Science News* says they are still dividing and are still in good health. We have discussed the research by Drs. Packer and Smith more fully in our chapter on aging.

The California scientists also performed experiments confirming the fact that **vitamin E, acting as a natural antioxidant, protects against certain air pollutants before they have a chance to damage cells**. They exposed cells treated with vitamin E and cells which had gotten no vitamin E. They exposed two kinds of cells to typical environmental stresses—oxygen and visible light. Of the cells which had obtained no vitamin E, 90 per cent were killed. Of those which had been given vitamin E, only 35 per cent died.

Says *Science News*, "On the basis of these findings

... Packer and Smith concluded that vitamin E is not a panacea for all aging processes. But they do believe that vitamin E will extend life where humans are subjected to severe environmental pollution. 'It might,' they speculate, 'prevent early death, or brain disease, heart attacks or senility.'"

An experiment that is significant for city dwellers who must breathe air pollution all day is reported in *Archives of Environmental Health* for May, 1975. Ozone is, say the authors, the most toxic element in air pollution. Ozone and nitrogen dioxide, another pollutant, react with unsaturated fatty acids in cells, resulting in damage to the cells. Giving laboratory rats vitamin E protects them from this damage.

Say the authors, all from Duke Medical Center in North Carolina, "Since the inhalation of ozone even at trace levels produces irreparable pulmonary (lung) injury in animals, direct experiments on man seem inappropriate." So they decided to test human blood cells which had been exposed to ozone and see if vitamin E in the diet of the person whose cells were tested made any difference.

It did. The volunteers who participated in the experiment were told to eat their usual diets. These contain, supposedly, about 8 milligrams of vitamin E daily. Blood was drawn from the volunteers and studied for the appearance of certain abnormal areas in the red blood cells which are caused by toxic agents—in this case, presumably ozone. Then the blood cells were exposed to ozone in the laboratory. Relatively low concentrations of ozone produced these unhealthy alterations in red blood cells.

Then the volunteers were given 100 milligrams of vitamin E daily for a week and more blood was taken and exposed to ozone. The number of disordered red blood cells had decreased noticeably. **In other words, it appeared that the vitamin E was protecting the cells from ozone damage**. The next week 200 milligrams of vitamin E were given daily. Some of the volunteers showed much greater protective action with the 200 milligrams. Others showed only a little.

The authors tell us that usually such disorders of red blood cells produce fatigue, very rapid heart beat and poor growth in children. No one knows apparently whether similar disorders induced by ozone in air pollutants produce the same effects. It seems likely that they may. **And it seems likely that vitamin E, perhaps up to 200 milligrams daily, may protect us from at least some of this damage**. Since these researchers used no more than 200 milligrams a day, we do not know whether perhaps even more vitamin E than that might protect completely from any damage at all to red blood cells.

The authors, cautious as most researchers are, refuse to speculate on whether the vitamin E actually protects the cells from damage. We see no reason to quibble or nit-pick. Vitamin E is harmless and inexpensive. Many people are taking it routinely for many reasons having to do with health. There seems to be no reason for not taking it if there is even a slight chance that it may help us survive the ever-present air pollution which we cannot escape.

We note that the Duke scientists feel it is "inappropriate" to subject human beings to experiments by exposing them to harmful levels of ozone. We wonder just what one would call daily life in a city where ozone in the air is inescapable. Isn't this an experiment on human beings? Aren't we all being experimented upon every day, so long as we must breathe such contaminated air?

The least we can do is to use every available weapon against the pollution, as well as complaining mightily to city, state and federal government officials, urging them to clean up urban air pollution no matter what the cost, before we have all expired or become chronically ill as a direct or indirect result of such pollution.

One other comment on this experiment. Officially we are told that adult men should have 15 milligrams or units of vitamin E daily, women should have 12 units. And, says the official body which decides these things, the "average

American diet" supplies this much vitamin E. Yet scientists in laboratories take for granted that their volunteers are getting no more than eight units of vitamin E daily and proceed on that basis. So it seems that most of us should be getting about twice the amount of vitamin E our diets give us, just to stay reasonably healthy, even without air pollution.

"Vitamins appear to play a much more vital role in safeguarding lungs from the ravages of air pollution than has been generally realized," says an article in *Chemical and Engineering News* for June 29, 1970. At a symposium on pollution and lung biochemistry at Battelle-Northwest Institute, a scientist from Massachusetts Institute of Technology told of his experiments with rats in which he found that the two fat-soluble vitamins—vitamin A and vitamin E—play an important role in protecting lung tissues from harm that may be done by two components of air pollution, ozone and nitrogen dioxide.

As indicated earlier, these two pollutants are among the most destructive compounds we have loosed on city dwellers from industrial pollution and the exhaust from automobiles that jam our city streets. Certain fatty substances in the lungs are broken down by the pollutants releasing other substances that are highly dangerous. **Vitamin E appears to "quench" these substances, rendering them harmless.**

Scientists from Battelle-Northwest have been conducting a series of nutrition experiments in which they fed rats a specially prepared diet that was high in polyunsaturates—the fatty substance which is attacked by the air pollutants. Some of the animals got food that contained no vitamin E. Others ate the same diet, supplemented with vitamin E.

The rats were then exposed to a stream of air containing one part per million of ozone. They soon showed signs of severe stress in breathing, and died. Those which were getting the vitamin E lived twice as long in the ozone-polluted atmosphere. In other experiments, researchers

84

autopsied the rats after they had been exposed to nitrogen dioxide. The animals that had eaten the diet deficient in vitamin E had far less of the polyunsaturates in their lungs than the rats which had plenty of vitamin E. Apparently the vitamin had preserved the valuable polyunsaturates and prevented their destruction.

Dr. Daniel B. Menzel, who heads the Battelle nutrition and food technology section, believes that **vitamin E might perform still another beneficial function in safeguarding vitamin A from being destroyed by the air pollutants**. "This in itself would be an important function," says the article, "because it is now becoming increasingly evident that vitamin A is crucial for the healthy metabolism and growth of epithelial cells." These are cells in the skin and linings of body cavities like the lungs.

At M.I.T. scientists have been experimenting with vitamin A, giving it to rats, then examining their lung cells. The rats which had plenty of vitamin A showed a healthy condition of the lungs. Those which had a deficiency showed cells that were thick, scaly and hard, instead of being soft and covered with healthful mucus. After identifying a certain compound present in the healthy lungs and absent in the deficient ones, they found furthermore that when they gave supplements of vitamin A to the deficient rats, this beneficial compound was formed in their lungs within 18 hours, even though they had been eating a deficient diet for a long time.

The researchers went on to say that we know now that vitamin A can prevent the formation of cells that later turn into cancer cells. They don't know exactly how the vitamin does this, but they are investigating the process. And now they are wondering whether massive doses of vitamin A may be able to reverse the growth of certain kinds of cancers. They are working with Dr. Umberto Saffiotti of the National Cancer Institute who has already proved that vitamin A, given orally to hamsters, can completely prevent the cancers that would normally appear when the animals are exposed to certain cancer-causing substances.

Environmental Research, Vol. 6, page 165, 1973, reported on experiments on laboratory rats exposed to toxic levels of ozone. **Vitamin E alone or in combination with other antioxidants exerted a protective effect.** Extracts of lung tissue from the rats which had been given the vitamin showed no damage to lungs. The rats not protected by the vitamin had pulmonary edema and hemorrhages which caused death.

Those animals given the largest amounts of antioxidants—1,500 milligrams each of vitamin E, plus vitamin C and methionine, an amino acid, showed the greatest survival rate. Ozone is one of the air pollutants common in large urban areas, as we have learned. A level of 0.8 parts per million of air approximates maximum levels for short periods during smog alerts in Los Angeles. Continuous exposure at this level resulted in death for all animals, even those protected by vitamin E.

The lesson seems clear. **If you live in an area of heavy air pollution, especially ozone, get lots and lots of vitamin E (1,500 milligrams each is an enormous dose for as small an animal as a rat).** And when a pollution alert goes out— leave town if you can. Get as far away as possible, for it seems that not even beneficent vitamin E is likely to protect you from a lengthy spell of such pollution.

CHAPTER 6

Vitamin E Is Important for a Successful Pregnancy

As FAR BACK as 1927 two scientists discovered that female laboratory rats which were kept on diets free of vitamin E could not successfully complete pregnancies, and male rats on such diets were sterile. This information has had very little effect on medically accepted treatment for lack of fertility in either male or female human beings.

All human beings get plenty of vitamin E in their diets, so there is no need to give them vitamin E to guarantee fertility—this seems to be the excuse for completely bypassing such a simple and harmless method of treatment. Apparently inquiry is seldom if ever made regarding the individual patient's intake of vitamin E. It is just assumed that lack of vitamin E could not possibly have anything to do with infertility in men or women.

Now we have another piece of evidence on the importance of this vitamin to fertility. Perhaps this, too, will be ignored, even though the experiment was supported financially by the National Institutes of Health, Public Health Service, and was described in an article in *Fertility and Sterility* for May-June, 1962.

Researchers in the laboratory at the University of Oregon had found that, although their female hamsters were fertile, the size of the litters was reduced as the animals grew older. The animals mated successfully and conceived as large litters as the younger animals. But, shortly before the end of pregnancy, some of the litters were "resorbed"— that is, they did not develop into baby hamsters, but were absorbed once again into the mother hamster. Laboratory animals are valuable for research, so it was considered worthwhile to discover how to prevent this from happening.

A group of older female hamsters were mated and then fed the usual laboratory diet during their pregnancy. This diet is not deficient in vitamin E incidentally. A second group of hamsters, which were also more than middle-aged, were mated and given the same diet plus 10 milligrams of vitamin E a day, in wheat germ oil.

Note the results. **Fifty-eight per cent of the females which had received the extra vitamin E successfully delivered litters, compared to only 23.4 per cent of the females which did not receive additional vitamin E.** Furthermore, the litters were larger in the first group, 5.20 animals as an average, whereas the second group, which did not receive the vitamin, had litters only about half as large.

Of the total number of females mated in the two groups, a relatively small number (16.1 per cent) of the vitamin-fed animals were infertile. Among those which got no extra vitamin E, 63.9 per cent were infertile.

The authors, Dr. A. L. Soderwall and Bryan C. Smith, conclude, "The data presented here, while not reflecting new ideas, do lend further support to the belief that certain nutritive substances enhance the probability of successful pregnancies in the mammalian female. The absence of adequate amounts of other vitamins, including vitamin A and some of the vitamin B group, have shown to be associated with fetal deaths or resorptions. It is interesting to note that the female does not seem to suffer too seriously and, indeed, may continue normal breeding behavior."

Animals in the group not fed vitamin E, which did not manage to deliver their young, suffered from varying degrees of hemorrhaging, indicating that the situation is about as it might be in a human abortion or miscarriage.

To confirm the need of vitamin E for successful pregnancies, the *Journal of the Palacky University* of Czechoslovakia, Vol. 25, 1961, contains an article on the vitamin E blood content of women. **The author found, among other things, that more than two-thirds of women tested who threatened to abort had decidedly less vitamin E in their blood than those who had normal pregnancies and deliveries**. It seems quite possible that the lack of the vitamin might have had a great deal to do with the condition—doesn't it?

A second confirmation of the relation of vitamin E to healthful pregnancy and childbirth occurs in *Obstetrics and Gynecology*, Vol. 20:1, 1962, in which Dr. D. G. McKay induced vitamin E deficiency in laboratory rats by feeding them diets low in the vitamin. These rats developed symptoms very much like symptoms of pregnancy toxemia, or poisoning, in human beings. Death in coma or convulsions, or death of the unborn young resulted. **Giving large amounts of vitamin E prevented these developments**.

An article in the Italian journal, *Minerva Ginecologia*, Vol. 13, page 1151, 1961, describes the injection of vitamin E into women just before childbirth. The vitamin E level in the blood of the new baby was then tested. There was no more than there would have been without the injection. These authors believe that the good effects of vitamin E are not involved just with labor. Only the administration of the vitamin during pregnancy can give the "brilliant results" reported previously. **This refers to the many, many accounts in foreign medical journals of vitamin E used successfully in pregnancy**.

A study of the amount of oxygen needed by the unborn child indicates that many things may lessen the supply of this important substance to the baby. An article in the *American Journal of Obstetrics and Gynecology*, Vol. 84, page 561, 1962, indicates that prolonged inhalation of an anesthetic may deprive the baby of oxygen. And toxemias of pregnancy—that is, serious states of illness during pregnancy—may deprive the baby of oxygen. Here again is the justification for using vitamin E during pregnancy because this vitamin has the unique ability to decrease the need for oxygen. **That is, the unborn child which is getting enough vitamin E will not need so much oxygen and so will not suffer so much from a reduced supply.**

Seven Canadian scientists reported in the *Canadian Journal of Physiology and Pharmacology* (3:384, 1974) that, in pregnancies ending in stillbirths, the vitamin E content of blood was lower than in normal pregnancies. Studies in animals indicate that a mother who is deficient in vitamin E is more likely to have congenital malformations in her offspring. The authors suggest that "the possibility of a vitamin basis for congenital deformities may be worth testing."

Two West German physicians reported in *Die Kapsel* in 1962 on many conditions helped by vitamin E: sterility, abortion, premature births and stillbirths, lactation troubles, menopause, disturbed menstruation, blood clots, angina pectoris, hardening of the arteries, ulcers, eczema, psoriasis and as an aid to insulin in diabetes. The dose of insulin can often be reduced when enough vitamin E is taken, they said.

In the December, 1972 issue of *The Summary*, edited by Dr. Evan Shute, it is reported that **vitamin E helps to prevent threatened abortion, premature rupture of membranes, prematurity and miscarriage**. In other references cited, vitamin E apparently had no effect on female sterility.

Concerning male sterility, 19 supportive medical papers

listed in *The Summary* indicate that **vitamin E improves the quality of the sperm cells, so fathers sire few or no congenitally damaged babies and their wives have fewer habitual abortions.**

As for non-eclamptic late toxemias, Dr. Shute said that vitamin E is no help in true eclampsia (convulsions or seizures associated with pregnancy) but in the non-convulsive or late type of this condition it is very helpful if used in time. Nineteen doctors have apparently found it so helpful that they have written medical papers on the subject.

A report in the Israeli journal, *Fertility and Sterility*, indicates that in 6 per cent of patients studied, the cause of abortion and miscarriage lay in the father's deficient sperm, not in any deficit of the mother's. The authors studied carefully the medical histories of many couples who had been married several times. Dr. Shute, reporting on this research in a 1966 issue of *The Summary*, said: "**We have long advocated alpha tocopherol (vitamin E) for poor sperm samples, especially in habitual abortion couples.**"

A Romanian farm journal reports that extremely large amounts of vitamin E, plus vitamin A, were given to 77 sterile cows. Within one to one and a half months, their sexual cycles were restored and 70 per cent of them conceived.

An important finding in relation to vitamin E is reported in *Science* for March 1, 1968. Two researchers at the University of California studied the process of reproduction in rats which had been deprived of vitamin E, although the rest of their diet was complete in every nutrient. They uncovered a very significant difference in the animals which got enough vitamin E and those which did not.

It is well known that sterility is the first indication of vitamin E deficiency in animals. Up to now, no one could even speculate why lack of vitamin E brought sterility. Scientists know that vitamin E is closely related in function to oxygen, in that it protects certain substances in food from oxidizing or becoming rancid. The two California scientists believe that this ability of vitamin E to protect substances from the action of oxygen may be necessary every time a cell divides. And, of course, cell division is the basis for reproduction and the growth of every new living thing.

Studying laboratory animals made deficient in vitamin E, the scientists found that their cells contained a given number of a certain particle in each cell that is not present in quantity when the cell is dividing normally. Animals which were getting plenty of vitamin E had fewer of these particles. They also found that animals raised breathing the regular air of the laboratory had a normal appearance, whereas the cells of those breathing pure oxygen looked more like the cells of animals which did not get enough vitamin E—another indication that too much oxygen was in some way damaging the process of cell division.

As the authors say in their article, they may have shown that vitamin E has the basic function of giving direct protection to the apparatus responsible for the division of cells. Now all cells divide, so this finding is not applicable only to problems of reproduction. The cells of children growing from infancy must divide many times to produce that growth. As we grow older, cells wear out and must be replaced by new cells.

Cancer is believed to be a disorder of cell division, where cells have lost the ability to limit their division and continue to divide wildly and profusely. So you can easily see what great importance may be attached to this finding in regard to vitamin E. If, indeed, ample amounts of this vitamin are essential to protect the apparatus whereby cells divide, then it is tied in indirectly with life itself and almost every process in life.

Of course, before we can make such a flat statement, other scientists in this field will have to confirm the work of the California researchers. Scientists in other fields will then have to relate this work to theirs before we finally have a definite scientific fact, accepted generally by most experts on nutrition. We do wish that the thousands of cancer researchers around the world would devote more experiments to vitamin E, rather than trying to develop a myriad of drugs, many of which have damaging side-effects. Vitamin E is harmless. But, as we know, the billion-dollar drug industries around the world make more money from new drugs than they do from using a relatively inexpensive vitamin like vitamin E.

In the latest issue of *The Summary*, published in 1977, an editorial in *The Lancet*, the British medical journal, is commented on.

The Lancet said there is a theory that there is such a thing as habitual abortion and there are frequent congenital abnormalities in the aborted fetuses. More and more, the thinking of the experts seems to indicate that inherited abnormalities may be responsible for most spontaneous abortions.

In women who have had a child with Down's Syndrome, for example, there is a 10 times greater than expected incidence of recurrent spontaneous abortions. Many of these may go unrecognized, says *The Lancet*. They may occur during one phase of the menstrual cycle without interrupting menstruation. Or they may occur a week or so later and not be recognized as an abortion.

Not more than 22 per cent of conceptions reach maturity. "Some of the women who abort repeatedly are first seen as problems in infertility," says *The Lancet*. They come to the doctor to see if he can suggest how they can become pregnant, while they are actually becoming pregnant over and over again and losing the baby at a very early stage of pregnancy.

The Shute Foundation editor comments at length on this theory. We think his comments should be very instructive. Many such women come to the Shute Foundation for Medical Research, the clinic in London, Ontario, Canada, and are surprised to find that they have symptoms of pregnancy without being pregnant. They may have colostrum in their breasts. They may remember some brief period in the past when a menstrual period was not exactly right, but it never occurred to them that they may have been pregnant. They may even have noticed nausea as well as tenderness and enlargement of the breasts. The Shutes believe that, in every such case, tests should be made for certain hormones in the womens' blood which will settle the matter.

And how do the Shutes treat this kind of spontaneous repeated abortion? With or without bed rest, they give vitamin E. And nothing else. They generally use from 75 to 100 units a day although, as they point out, there is no reason not to give much more—up to 800 units, if necessary. And larger doses may seem wise if the patient is "spotting" blood. "Some bleedings of considerable amount can thus be controlled," they say. The most reliable way to make a diagnosis of pregnancy or no pregnancy is to give vitamin E in these dosages and then continue to examine the woman from time to time to see if her uterus is enlarging.

The Shutes believe, too, that in order to prevent miscarriages and spontaneous abortions, it is wise to give vitamin E to the baby's father before conception in the hope of getting the very best possible sperm cell and the best possible egg cell to start out the new life and give it enough vigor to resist stress that might cause spontaneous abortion.

"We have long believed and reported that this is the most effective way of treating recurrent abortions, since early pregnancies are so often unrecognized. **A woman with a bad abortion history should probably take vitamin E for years on end in the hope of securing the best possible nidation (implantation in the uterus) to an ovum at the stage when it might still be unrecognized and tend to be expelled without symptoms,"** the Shutes report.

Dr. Evan Shute is one of Canada's most distinguished

obstetricians. It seems to us that this simple, inexpensive method of preventing abortion mishaps should be undertaken by every young woman who is planning to become pregnant, and every young man who fathers the child.

A letter to the editor in the May, 1975 issue of the *American Journal of Clinical Nutrition* comes from Michael and Maxine Briggs of Melbourne, Australia, who say there is excellent and compelling evidence that **oral contraceptives (The Pill) have deleterious effects on the body's store of vitamin E**. It lowers blood levels of the vitamin and increases individual dietary requirements for it.

The two Dr. Briggs studied 15 healthy young women just starting to take The Pill. Before they began, the concentration of vitamin E in their blood was approximately 14 milligrams per liter. After they had taken The Pill for three months, the vitamin E concentration was about 11 milligrams.

They then gave the women vitamin E daily to see how much was necessary to bring the levels back to where they were before The Pill was started. The women needed supplements of 10 milligrams daily to achieve this. The Australian physicians speculate on what effects lack of vitamin E may eventually have on the circulatory health of young women on The Pill. It is known that they are more likely to suffer from strokes and other circulatory complications. Could these be caused by lack of vitamin E brought about by The Pill?

CHAPTER 7

What's Wrong When Healthy Babies Suddenly Die?

"IN THE MIDDLE of October (1976), we took our baby, Amaris, to her first political rally to hear Jimmy Carter. On October 20, we celebrated her one-year-old birthday party. On October 31, we took her 'trick or treating.' On November 2, we took her along when we went to vote. On November 14, we took her to the cemetery to say good-by."

So began the testimony of a Belvedere, California father who was one of 19 witnesses to appear before the Senate Human Resources subcommittee, which held hearings in March, 1978 on crib death or Sudden Infant Death Syndrome (SIDS). This tragic story was retold in a press release issued by Senator Alan Cranston (D., Calif.) who has introduced a bill to appropriate more money for research into the causes and treatment of crib death.

First recognized as a distinct disorder less than 10 years ago, **crib death is today the single largest cause of death among infants between the ages of one month and one year**. It kills perhaps 20,000 American babies every year. This cruel drama takes its toll of young parents as well, many of whom are unjustly suspected of being responsible for the baby's death. Many of the parents also assume unwarranted guilt and blame themselves, thinking they must have done something wrong.

The perfectly healthy baby is put to bed, cooing and smiling. His mother comes to check on him during the night, or the next morning, and finds him dead, with no sign of a struggle or any convulsive movements. Physicians and researchers have suggested many causes. Most of them seem to be related to the completely unnatural conditions that surround most American babies from the very moment of birth.

Dr. Mavis Gunther, a British physician, theorizes in the February 22, 1975 issue of *The Lancet* that "cot deaths" as they are called in England, result from infections or allergies induced in the baby by bottle-feeding. Her reasoning is that all mammalian young refuse any kind of food except their mother's milk during an appropriate period after birth. It is well known to scientists that breast milk contains resistance factors which protect the baby from infections until he is old enough to develop his own protective mechanism.

"The effectiveness of breast feeding in defense against viral and bacterial infection has only tardily been accepted, but it is real," says Dr. Gunther. **The first milk after childbirth, called colostrum, is known to be very rich in protective factors, but so, too, is breast milk later on.** Certainly bottle-fed babies are more liable to infection. Some pediatricians believe this is because the mechanics of bottle-feeding lend themselves to contamination with bacteria. But in animals as well as human beings vital protection against an array of disorders is guaranteed by mother's milk, whereas cow's milk contains no such protection for human babies.

Rabbits that are raised in germ-free environments and fed on cow's milk die when they are 18 to 22 days old, says Dr. Gunther, at an age when behavior ordinarily makes mammary feeding obligatory and nibbling on other food is only starting. In the case of the rabbits, as in human babies, death may be caused by bacteria to which the infant has not developed immunity or to some allergen to which he is susceptible.

Most babies which die of crib death are bottle-fed. The risk is much greater also in babies whose weight at birth was too low. The incidence is much higher, too, among young mothers who had had children in quick succession without access to highly nutritious diets. **So lack of protein and lack of folic acid, a B vitamin, are suspected as one more reason for such tragedies.** Babies dying this way generally have watery accumulations in their lungs, suggesting that they could not get enough oxygen to keep breathing normally.

In the same issue of *The Lancet* comes word from another British source that **lack of vitamin E and the trace mineral selenium may have something to do with crib deaths.** Vitamin E does not pass freely from mother to unborn baby, say Drs. E. Tapp and C. Anfield of Manchester. Human babies are born with much lower levels of vitamin E in their blood than adults have. They may develop a kind of anemia as a result. The levels of vitamin E in the blood rise much more slowly in infants given formulas than in those who are breast-fed. **A study of 14 infants dying of crib death showed in general much lower levels of vitamin E than in those babies who died of other conditions.**

And from New Zealand, in November, 1971, evidence reached us from an Animal Health Laboratory that human babies are being raised under conditions of deficiency in both selenium and vitamin E, which would not for a moment be tolerated in animal husbandry. Says Dr. F. C. Money, autopsies of the victims of crib death show the same conditions found in animals dead from lack of vitamin E and the trace mineral selenium. "Many fatal vitamin E and/or selenium deficiency diseases of the young of about 40 mammalian and bird species are known," he says. Most deaths occur only when both nutrients are lacking, since one can substitute for the other.

Found at autopsies are hemorrhages from small blood vessels in the lungs and adjacent chest walls, filling of the lungs with blood fluid, degenerative changes of, and hemorrhages in the vital heart muscle and hemorrhages around the spinal cord. When there is not enough oxygen, Dr. Money says, "the normal oxidative processes by which tissues gain their energy and heat, extend into the tissues themselves where chain reaction proceeds unchecked. Simply this means that otherwise healthy tissues combust. The reaction is termed peroxidation and in prevention of this vitamin E acts as an antioxidant."

Dr. Money goes on to describe other conditions of infants, such as *retrolental fibroplasia*, **which causes blindness which can be prevented by vitamin E.** This disorder occurred in many premature infants exposed to too high a concentration of oxygen in their incubators, long before anyone suspected what was causing these tragedies.

Consumer Bulletin for June, 1972 tells us that cow's milk is deficient in vitamin E and high in phosphates, which the baby's kidneys have trouble dealing with. **In human milk there is considerably more vitamin E and it is in proper balance with the unsaturated fats.** This is important, since getting too much of these fats tends to raise one's needs for vitamin E. The *Bulletin* tells us that guinea pigs fed a diet deficient in vitamin E showed many of the same conditions, after death, that infants dying of crib death show.

A disease of newborn infants called Respiratory Distress Syndrome may be caused by lack of lecithin in their lungs, according to a group of Welsh physicians who reported their findings in *Nature* for February 25, 1972. This is a disease which kills babies within a few days after birth. Tests on 97 infants showed that those who were delivered in good health had lecithin levels of 3.5 to 37.5. Of

13 infants who developed the respiratory disease, lecithin levels were only 0.6 to 3.4. In every case the lowest level of lecithin accompanied the most severe respiratory distress.

Breast milk is a mixture of many things, including lecithin and cholesterol, as well as trace minerals, B vitamins, vitamin A, vitamin C and the minerals calcium and phosphorus. Now we learn that it contains much larger amounts of vitamin E than does cow's milk. Everyone who makes official statements in the field of pediatrics admits that no one can reproduce breast milk, no matter how hard they try. It's simply too complex a mixture, so there is no way of knowing how many other essential elements we are leaving out when we mix up formula or feed the baby already mixed formulas.

The New Zealand veterinary physician, as long ago as 1972, was calling for infant formulas fortified with vitamin E to prevent more crib deaths. Of course he believed, as do all other workers in this field, that breast milk is the ideal food for infants. **But if breast-feeding is impossible, then certainly baby's formula should contain at least as much vitamin E as is present in breast milk.**

Time and again in experiments and experiences dealing with animals, we run across the flat statement that vitamin E in considerable amounts is absolutely essential for good health in this or that species of bird or animal—chickens, dogs, race horses, guinea pigs. Such animals are valuable. Their health is the urgent concern of the people who own them and who pay vast sums of money to keep them healthy. Everybody involved in caring for such valuable animals agrees that they should have access to every nutrient that they can utilize for supernutrition. Horse, chicken and dog feed is well fortified with vitamin E, since its value for a healthy sex and reproductive life has been assured, as well as its value for preventing heart and circulatory disorders and many related conditions.

But when it comes to human beings, we are told officially that all Americans automatically get enough vitamin E in their food, even though every official survey shows that most of us simply do not eat those foods in which vitamin E is most abundant: whole grains, raw seeds and nuts and foods made from them like wholegrain breads and cereals, plus seed and cereal oils like corn, safflower, soybean and peanut oil which, being concentrated foods, contain the most vitamin E.

People who neglect salads get almost no salad oils. If they don't eat mayonnaise, eggs, leafy green vegetables like spinach, parsley and watercress, they are neglecting vitamin E. **If they always eat white bread and supermarket processed cereals they are getting almost no vitamin E.** Officially an adult needs up to 15 milligrams daily. The best sources are salad oils, wheat germ, wheat bran, whole seeds of all kinds, wholegrains, eggs, leafy vegetables, legumes such as peas, beans and lentils, liver, meat, milk and peanuts. **Up to 90 per cent of the vitamin E is lost during the processing of supermarket cereals.** Many scientists feel certain vitamin E should be added to all such foods.

And an increasingly large number of physicians believe it is healthy to get much more vitamin E than the official recommendation: two or three hundred milligrams or perhaps more for good health, especially if you have circulatory problems.

For those who wish more information about breast-feeding, write to: La Leche League, 9616 Minneapolis Avenue, Franklin Park, Illinois 60131.

For more information about the birth of healthy children rather than children with low birth weight and other congenital defects, write to: Society for the Protection of the Unborn Through Nutrition, SPUN, 17 North Wabash Avenue, Suite 603, Chicago, Illinois 60602.

Vitamin C can also be important in possibly preventing crib deaths, according to information we learned after listening to the tape of an Australian radio program on the subject of infant and baby health.

The doctors who spoke in Australia believe that lack of

vitamin C may be largely responsible for crib death, combined with the extra stress on the child from the numerous immunizations which are customarily given very young infants. Dr. Archie Kalokerinos told of Aborigine babies in the Australian area where he practices medicine. He was horrified when he came to the area to discover that one out of every two Aborigine babies was dying from unknown causes very early in life. All the babies and children brought to him suffered almost constantly from runny noses, infected ears and coughs. Gastrointestinal diseases and pneumonia were commonplace. They occurred in the same children. It was evident that the children were badly nourished and lived under unhygienic conditions. So Dr. Kalokerinos gave them antibiotics and the customary vitamin supplements.

He says, in his startling book on the subject, *Every Second Child*, "If it was known that the diet included, for example, 30 milligrams of vitamin C ... a day then there seemed no reason for concern. ... Much had been written about this vital subject and an enormous amount of research had been done. One leading research institute after another had clearly demonstrated that under conditions of stress, infections and injury there was an increased utilization of vitamin C and 30 milligrams a day may not be sufficient to cope with the increased demand." But this information had been ignored by the medical profession and even dedicated physicians like Dr. Kalokerinos had not heard of this research.

When he did hear about it, Dr. Kalokerinos brought these tragic figures on child mortality down to zero by simply giving all the babies who were brought to him enough vitamin C to prevent any deficiency, no matter how great was the stress to which the child was exposed and how great the child's need for the vitamin. The photographs in his book show babies brought in with tender limbs, irritability, "running" ears, teething problems—all desperately needing much more vitamin C than they had been

102

getting. And there are pictures of the babies relaxed, sleepy and smiling after injection of vitamin C.

Speaking of crib deaths, Dr. Kalokerinos says, "Some sudden unexpected deaths occur in infants who appear to be perfectly well, do not suffer from illnesses of any sort, are placed in a cot to rest or sleep and are later found dead. Mostly no cause is found and these are typical cases. I hesitate before stating that all these typical cases are due to vitamin C deficiency. Some definitely are. It is possible that they all are . . . often death is not really sudden. An infant may appear to be mildly ill, then suddenly collapse, become shocked and die. The variation of the infant's requirements for vitamin C are tremendous. Adults do not exhibit this. Adult scurvy is therefore a slow process."

One possible cause of the baby's greatly increased need for vitamin C is the immunization program which, in Australia as in our country, is almost mandatory for very young infants. Dr. Kalokerinos noticed that crib deaths and other unexplained deaths were more frequent in winter (when fresh foods rich in vitamin C were unavailable) and during and after immunization programs. There seems to be no doubt that immunization for childhood diseases is a form of great stress. This means that the baby's needs for vitamin C increase greatly. If no provision is made for this by increasing the baby's intake of vitamin C, a condition resembling scurvy or scurvy itself will probably follow.

Many of the children Dr. Kalokerinos treated had no visible symptoms of vitamin C deficiency. Others had the aching bones, the irritability, the swollen gums which any old-time doctor would have recognized as scurvy. But modern physicians have been convinced that all babies get plenty of vitamin C in their formulas or in fruit juices, so they do not anticipate any scurvy symptoms, nor look for them.

Dr. Fred Klenner of North Carolina, who uses massive doses of vitamin C to treat many disorders, spoke on the Australian radio program. He is a specialist in chest and respiratory diseases. He said that any child with nasal congestion is a likely candidate for crib death. He gives all infants and children in his care up to one gram (1,000 milligrams) of vitamin C daily. He said that any doctor who tries it will discover that vitamin C, in proper amounts, will destroy a virus within 96 minutes or less, especially if the vitamin is injected. Victims of crib death die from suffocation, he said. He prescribes one-half to one gram of vitamin C every hour, if the child with a respiratory disease has a temperature less than 100 degrees. If it is over that, he gives the vitamin by injection.

Mothers ask him why babies die in bed rather than during the day. They are put to bed with stuffed nostrils, he says, resulting from respiratory infections, however slight. They die of suffocation. By destroying the infectious virus you prevent the nasal stuffiness. Mothers should also clean mucus from any infant's nostrils very carefully before putting the child to bed, if any evidence of colds or nasal stuffiness is present.

Other physicians on the program told of finding many infants with no vitamin C at all in their urine. One doctor said that one mother out of every 24 that he treats has no vitamin C in her breast milk. Australian babies are given a formula called "Sunshine milk" which contains no vitamin C. If babies of mothers who are also deficient in vitamin C are given no vitamin supplements containing this essential substance, they will surely suffer from lack of the vitamin which is used in many body processes, which is easily and rapidly excreted and easily destroyed by many toxins.

Cigarette smoke, for example. The prospective mother who smokes will surely have no vitamin C to pass along to her unborn baby since smoking destroys vitamin C wholesale in our bodies. The child who grows up in a house where the air is thick with cigarette smoke is getting almost as much exposure to this toxin as adults are, and, since he is so much smaller, the effects on him are probably much more serious.

"125 crib death infants, followed from birth, were compared to a similar group of living babies," reported *American Journal of Diseases of Children*, November, 1976. "Some of the crib death victims showed evidence of brain dysfunction including abnormalities in breathing, feeding and temperature regulation. More of the dead infants had been born to mothers who smoked and had anemia."

Homeostasis Quarterly is published by the Adrenal Metabolic Research Society of the Hypoglycemia Foundation. Its Summer, 1975 issue dealt with crib death. Here is a quote:

"The *New York Times*, July 5, 1975 carried a report on the findings of Dr. Henry Lardy, Wisconsin University Enzyme Institute, pointing to a defect in amino acid (protein) metabolism with resulting low blood sugar levels, as a possible cause of sudden infant death. Dr. Lardy observed, if a baby's ability to synthesize sugar is not efficient, as long as he is fed every few hours, he is fine. However, during a long fast, sleeping through the night, for instance, or missing a feeding, the blood sugar may fall extremely low and the baby may not be able to convert amino acids efficiently with resulting fatal hypoglycemia (low blood sugar). It was pointed out, in addition, that a number of babies, victims of SID, had a history of 'fits' and fits are a classic symptom of low blood sugar. Dr. Lardy presented his report at the First Annual Workshop on Sudden Infant Death Syndrome, sponsored by the National Institutes of Health.

"Sudden Infant Death Syndrome is a tragic situation, one which is well understood by the editor of *Homeostasis*, who lost her only child in this fashion 18 years ago. Numbers of theories have been put forward as to the cause. Now there is a breakthrough. Inefficient blood sugar regulation dominates the scene. Pertinent is a report on clinical aspects of hypoglycemia in newborn infants (Fluge, G., *Acta Paediat. Scand.* 63:826, 1974). Dr. Fluge stresses the need for blood glucose (sugar) determinations in ALL infants, pointing out those at particular risk are infants born to mothers who had toxemia of pregnancy and infants, full-term, but low birth weight." For a copy of this very significant article in full, write to the Society named above, at P.O. Box 98, Fleetwood, Mt. Vernon, N. Y. 10552.

A new book on *Crib Death* by Richard H. Raring discusses just about everything that is known officially about this epidemic disaster, including a chapter on *Theories and Research* in which he touches on the subject of vitamins and other diet deficiencies. Mr. Raring had apparently not heard of the Australian research when he wrote his book, for he dismisses Dr. Klenner's use of vitamin C in massive doses as "one more theory, neither proven, disproven nor tested."

This brings us to a realization of the fact that crib death, like cancer, may have a multitude of manifestations and a multitude of causes. So far orthodox medical science has turned up nothing which gives parents any hope that their baby can escape this terrible fate. It seems to us that any intelligent parent, faced with the facts, must realize that giving vitamins to a baby is no more difficult and no more risky than giving him food and water. So why quibble about whether the "theories" on low blood sugar, vitamin C and vitamin E are just "theories" or whether they can be useful in preventing this tragedy? Let the scientists and researchers quibble and nitpick! They go through this procedure with every new idea that appears in the realm of health, disease and medicine, especially if vitamins are involved. But meanwhile give your baby whatever chance for a healthy life you can give him by using whatever helpful information you can find—including the well-documented facts from Dr. Kalokerinos and Dr. Klenner as well as the article in *Homeostasis*.

Vitamin E is the nutrient quite likely to be deficient in modern baby formulas, according to two University of

106

Wyoming scientists writing in the *American Journal of Clinical Nutrition*, March, 1967. Drs. Martha Dicks-Bushnell and Karen Davis tested baby formulas for vitamin E and found that the processing through which the formulas go tends to destroy their vitamin E content.

Babies fed on six commercial formulas and 10 baby cereals seemed to have a deficiency in vitamin E, while those who were breast-fed showed an increase in vitamin E content of their blood. The doctors recommended that all baby formulas should be supplemented with vitamin E.

The official booklet, *Recommended Dietary Allowances*, 1974, states that babies should receive in their food the amount of vitamin E that is present in human milk. This same book mentions many of the conditions of ill-health that appear to have some relation to vitamin E deficiency: some blood disorders, cystic fibrosis, encephalo-malacia, certain kinds of cirrhosis, celiac disease, sprue and other disorders. Could it be that the increasing incidence of these conditions may have something to do with modern infants not getting enough of this important vitamin in their formulas?

Vitamin E is available in liquid preparations, easy to include in baby's formula. Of course, the best food for infants is mother's milk, and there appears abundant evidence that no breast-fed baby will be deficient in vitamin E or any other essential. But for those who are unable to nurse their infants, it seems wise to include a vitamin E supplement from the beginning.

The books referred to above are:

Every Second Child by Archie Kalokerinos, available from the Book Department at Bronson Pharmaceuticals, 2546 Rinetti Lane, La Canada, California 91011. Price, $8.10.

Crib Death by Richard H. Raring, published by Exposition Press, Inc., 900 South Oyster Bay Road, Hicksville, N. Y. 11801 for $6.50.

CHAPTER 8

Premature Babies and Vitamin E

PREMATURE BABIES are born with very low levels of vitamin E, say Janet E. Graeber and her colleagues, writing in the February, 1977 issue of *The Journal of Pediatrics*. Giving the babies formulas in which there is a lot of unsaturated fats (from vegetable oils) tends to make this deficiency worse, since the more unsaturated fats one gets in food the more vitamin E is needed. Giving iron supplements by mouth to the babies also makes the deficiency worse, since iron medications are, generally speaking, destructive of vitamin E.

Dr. Graeber and her colleagues tested the blood of a group of 35 "preemies." Some of these were getting vitamin E supplements. And some of them were getting iron by mouth. Others got iron injections. Dr. Graeber found that giving large doses of vitamin E (125 to 150 milligrams per two pounds) improved the blood picture and resulted in satisfactory levels of vitamin E in all the children. In those who got the iron injections, vitamin E levels went up satisfactorily. **But babies getting iron by mouth and no vitamin E supplements showed the worst blood condition.**

It is in the digestive tract that iron medication interferes with absorption of vitamin E. When iron is given by injection, this does not occur. This is the reason we suggest that, if you are taking iron medication, you time your vitamin E intake as far as possible from the time you take your iron pills. Take one in the morning, the other at night, for example.

Dr. Graeber points out that *signs of anemia due to vitamin E deficiency are serious in "preemies" and we must also consider that other unrecognized damage may be done to the infant due to lack of vitamin E.* For instance, some years ago premature babies were routinely given oxygen to help in breathing. Later many of these children became blind from a disease called *retrolental fibroplasia.* So oxygen is not administered now. Could not part of the difficulty have been lack of vitamin E, Dr. Graeber asks.

The anemia for which she was testing the babies is a late manifestation of prolonged vitamin E deficiency, she says. But injury to other tissues may have occurred earlier and gone unnoticed. She believes, she says, that pediatricians and obstetricians should give thought to giving premature babies routine injections of vitamin E very early, to prevent any damage that might occur from lack of this antioxidant substance.

As long ago as 1974, the classical volume *Vitamins and Hormones* presented the same evidence of **damage to premature infants due to vitamin E deficiency.** Dr. J. Marks states in this volume that it is now agreed that all premature infants who are getting formulas rich in unsaturated fats should also get supplements of 10 milligrams of vitamin E per day right from the tenth day after birth. Children who have problems digesting fats should be getting 100 milligrams of the vitamin daily, says Dr. Marks.

Retinitis pigmentosa is an eye disease, supposedly hereditary, which may be initiated by vitamin E deficiency, says Dr. Marks. Giving about 100 milligrams of vitamin E daily, along with vitamin A, has prevented further deterioration in this condition, which usually leads to blindness.

In intermittent claudication, a condition of adults in which it is impossible to walk because of excruciating pain in the legs, "sustained high dosage" of vitamin E is necessary to alleviate this condition. This means, says Dr. Marks, doses which may be 20 to 30 times the normal daily requirements. Should one take daily supplements of vitamin E? Yes, says Dr. Marks, especially if there is any condition of the intestine which might make absorption of fats unreliable. This would, we imagine, involve just about any disorder of the intestine.

Getting back to premature infants, we know that **some modern formulas for babies are very high in the unsaturated fats, which would increase the need for vitamin E.** We know, too, that the milk given to grossly premature babies is usually very low in this protective substance. Vitamin E does not pass through the placental barrier from the pregnant mother to the infant she carries, so most babies are born vitamin E-deficient.

If the baby has the usual birth weight and is not premature, the mother's milk and formula usually correct this deficiency by the end of the first week of life. In the premature baby, however, the deficiency is more pronounced and persistent, according to two Welch physicians, writing in *International Journal of Vitamin Research*, Vol. 40, 1970. Dr. M. A. Chadd and A. J. Fraser review the evidence and then tell us about their own experience with premature infants.

They followed the course of 52 infants, some of whom were given vitamin E supplements, others not. No matter what their weight at birth was, all the infants getting vitamin E showed higher blood levels of vitamin E within a week, demonstrating that there was no problem with absorbing the vitamin. And at the usual time when anemia is expected to appear, **the babies who got vitamin E showed higher blood levels of iron than those which did not.**

In the case of premature babies, whose birth weight was

very low, the vitamin E made no difference in the tendency to anemia. The doctors feel that perhaps they were not giving enough of the vitamin. They stress the fact that more work needs to be done to determine what amounts of the vitamin will be most beneficial, depending on the baby's weight. They think that the premature ones may have a worse deficiency than the normal ones, hence may need much more of the vitamin.

In a second article in the same journal, they tell us of three babies who were "grossly immature" and suffering from symptoms of vitamin E deficiency. They were swollen and suffered from anemia. They had received routine supplements of vitamins, iron and folic acid, a B vitamin, but the condition persisted. They were given 12 milligrams of vitamin E and responded immediately. The swelling went down, the blood picture improved at once.

Say the authors, "It is suggested that **vitamin E deficiency be considered in any very small infant who has an anemia within a few weeks of birth.**"

These researchers do not discuss the diet of the mothers of these children. But if the vitamin E does not pass readily from mother to unborn child, does it not seem possible that this may be because of lack of vitamin E in the mother? Many researchers have shown that modern diets, in which refined foods make up a large part, are lacking in this vitamin. Is it not possible that these infants' mothers were just not getting enough of it to pass some along to the babies?

Considering the close relationship of vitamin E to reproductive functions, isn't it possible, too, that **lack of vitamin E in the mother's diet may be one of the main reasons for the babies being born prematurely?** Veterinarians have known for years that horses and prize animals of many kinds are liable to abort their young or to deliver them prematurely when they are short on vitamin E. Many stock raisers use the vitamin regularly to prevent this condition. Too bad many of our human children are not

111

given the benefit of this beneficent vitamin as valuable stock animals are.

The Summary for 1966, edited by Dr. Evan Shute, reports that animals deficient in vitamin E produced young with gross and microscopic defects of the skeleton, muscles and nervous system. They had harelips, abdominal hernias, badly curved backs and many more defects. This research appeared originally in *The Journal of Animal Science*, Vol. 22, page 848, 1963.

From the same edition of *The Summary*, two American obstetricians report in the *American Journal of Obstetrics and Gynecology* that they know of no way to prevent serious damage and death for many premature infants. Dr. Shute comments, "These authors apparently have not seen our reports on the use of alpha tocopherol (vitamin E) in the prevention of prematurity." He goes on to say, "No comparable results have ever been reported."

In another issue of *The Summary*, which contains abstracts, reports, letters and other documents from doctors around the world concerning vitamin E, Dr. Shute himself reported on vitamin E preventing premature births in 1954. He writes, with characteristic vigor, "the interest (among physicians) is very vague and until recently has concentrated on the care of the puny newborn as if prematurity itself were an unavoidable Act of God, perhaps occurring when the Creator was too drowsy to keep track of His Clock." Dr. Shute gives vitamin E, with success in 76 per cent of the patients he reports on here.

He also tells of three Hungarian physicians, who gave **"massive doses of natural vitamin E to infants with acute thrombophlebitis, with excellent results."** They have had similar good results giving it to adults with chronic thrombophlebitis.

An editorial in the *British Medical Journal* in 1974 (Vol. 2, page 625) discussed the power of vitamin E in maintaining the membrane of red blood cells. Low levels of vitamin E put circulating red cells "at risk," says the editorial. **Children not getting enough protein or vitamin E may suffer from a kind of anemia caused by these two deficiencies.** Protein alone does not cure the condition. Vitamin E must be given. Premature infants may suffer from this anemia which results from lack of vitamin E. Treatment with iron seems to worsen the condition.

The *Journal* reports that lack of vitamin E may be a major feature of the disease called *thalassemia*. This is a kind of anemia most common among Greek people which is believed to be hereditary. One would think that an hereditary disease could not be treated with a vitamin. But giving vitamin E to six patients restored the red blood cells in every case.

A Yale professor of pediatrics recently reported to a National Foundation-sponsored conference that giving oxygen to premature babies can produce lung damage. The respirators from which the babies breathe high concentration oxygen bring about reduced lung function after about a day. Too much oxygen seems to oxidize fatty elements in the lung membranes. This can lead to lung failure and heart damage.

Injecting vitamin E seems to protect the infants from harm, for the vitamin E seems to "sit in the membrane" and collect the damaging oxygen, according to *Medical World News*.

A second problem with premature babies on oxygen, as we stated earlier, has always been the very serious eye condition called retrolental fibroplasia. The unborn baby's retina grows naturally in the amount of oxygen provided in the mother's womb. A premature baby must adapt to oxygen tensions of the hospital room in which it is placed. So it is given oxygen to prevent damaged retinas which, in the past, led to many cases of blindness.

At the University of Pennsylvania hospital, **Dr. Lois Johnson has been giving vitamin E orally to prematures to protect against retinal damage.** Although her chief interest lies in protecting the babies' eyes, she says she has noted an improvement in the babies' breathing problems when vitamin E is given. She thinks vitamin E therapy will be important even for premature babies who do not need oxygen. Says *Medical World News*, reporting on this in the October 3, 1977 issue, "Since there are no apparent ill effects of the therapy, Dr. Johnson advocates giving oral vitamin E to preemies as soon as possible after birth. . . ."

In July, 1975, *Nutrition Reviews* discussed the prevention of peroxides (or rancidity) in cells of premature babies by the use of vitamin E. **In infants who are deficient in vitamin E, red blood cells suffer a disabling condition which results in anemia for the baby.**

As previously indicated, premature babies are more at risk than those born at term for they come into the world with less vitamin E stores in their bodies and their capacity to absorb the vitamin is less than that of normal infants.

The *British Medical Journal* for October 4, 1975 told of a 16-month-old infant with liver trouble, chronic jaundice and gall bladder trouble, who was also found to be deficient in vitamin E. A study of his blood revealed that blood cells were abnormal in a fashion that suggested vitamin E deficiency. **Giving the vitamin completely corrected the blood disorder.**

In the case of premature infants, they must have oxygen therapy or they will die. Giving them oxygen therapy may bring on the serious eye condition called *retrolental fibroplasia* which may cause blindness. Fifteen years ago this disaster was striking premature infants in epidemic proportions, says *Medical World News* for September 13, 1974. Today doctors have many new methods for preventing the eye disorder, but these improvements have not eliminated the problem. Conditions such as severe myopia (short-sightedness), strabismus (crossed eyes), amblyopia (dimness of vision) and other conditions may develop even if the child does not become permanently blind.

Three Philadelphia physicians, working on the problem, asked themselves whether vitamin E might not help out, since it is known as an antioxidant. That is, it protects foods from oxidation or becoming rancid. It also protects body cells from possible harmful effects of too much oxygen. Is it not possible, said Drs. Lois Johnson, David Schaffer and Thomas R. Boggs, that vitamin E might protect premature infants from the harmful effects of oxygen, given to prevent the eye disease (RLF) which causes blindness. They noted, too, **that many premature babies are deficient in vitamin E.**

Working with 81 children all of whom were premature and had very small birth weights, they gave 41 of these babies vitamin E injections from the first hours of life until the eye tissues most sensitive to RLF had completely matured or until any active disease had disappeared. They maintained blood levels of the vitamin in this group of babies. The other 40 infants received no vitamin E.

In 22 per cent of the treated infants some degree of retrolental fibroplasia occurred, but the non-treated children had a much higher incidence of 37.5 per cent. The children treated with vitamin E also had much better scores on severity of disease and the actual number of eyes affected. Among children who developed RLF, 15½ weeks passed before the disease disappeared, if they had received no vitamin E. But children who got the vitamin were disease-free in six weeks.

Following up the children for one year, the physicians found that **the condition of the vitamin E-treated babies was better.** A veteran specialist in the disease said that vitamin E therapy is still too experimental to be an everyday part of treatment, but the Philadelphia physicians have "charted a sound course." So still another experiment shows **the close relation between vitamin E and oxygen.**

In *The American Journal of Clinical Nutrition* for September, 1972, Karen C. Davis of the Agricultural

Experiment Station, University of Idaho, tells us about the amount of vitamin E in baby's diets in the United States.

As might be expected, **she found that the situation in regard to vitamin E in commercial baby food is chaotic, completely chaotic.** Since American parents spent $344,700,000 for baby foods every year, it is apparent that most babies are fed out of drug store bottles and supermarket cartons. Breast feeding being generally considered too inconvenient, most babies live on formulas which are bought at the store. It's also too inconvenient to prepare baby's formula at home apparently.

Because of the nationwide scare over cholesterol, commercial baby's formulas these days are loaded with unsaturated fats, rather than good, old saturated fat that comes in human milk and cow's milk. But unsaturated fats must be accompanied by very sizable amounts of vitamin E or they create a deficiency in this vitamin. And most of the commercial formulas Dr. Davis studied contained little or no vitamin E.

So, in consultation with a local pediatrician, she designed complete all-day feeding schedules for babies of different ages using 23 different commercial formulas, plus fruit, cereal and vegetables. And she carefully calculated the amount of vitamin E the infants might get from such diets. She found that the minimum amount of vitamin E was 1.38 milligrams, the maximum was 14.92 milligrams, depending on which formulas were used!

She came to the conclusion that the range of vitamin E varies so greatly that **"it becomes a matter of real concern to choose formulas and foods that are adequate with respect to both vitamin E and the ratio of vitamin E to the unsaturated fats . . . Baby foods generally do not supply much vitamin,"** she says, mostly because the cereals are all refined cereals, and fruits and vegetables are not very good sources of the vitamin. So, she says, we should fortify the commercial formulas with vitamin E. Some of them are already fortified, but probably have too little of the

116

vitamin.

Interestingly enough, whenever cereal appears on her list of foods, the infant always gets one teaspoon of sugar, plain white sugar, along with the cereal—just to make sure, we guess, that the child will be addicted to sugar by the time he can toddle. Or maybe pediatricians and nutritionists simply do not know that children have no need of added sugar, and don't especially like it but very soon become addicted to the taste. Adults apparently go right on assuming that babies are born with the same perverted sense of taste their parents have developed, over the years, in regard to sugar and salt.

What to do? We suggest, if there's a new baby at your home, that breast-feeding is infinitely superior to any formula and that all babies should be breast-fed as long as possible. We also suggest that homemade formulas are infinitely superior to commercial ones, that they should be made of cow's milk or goat milk diluted to make them as nearly identical to human breast milk as possible and that early foods should include cooked cereals with as much vitamin E as possible, as well as egg yolk and pureed meat along with fruits and vegetables.

For more information on breast feeding, write to: La Leche League, 9616 Minneapolis Avenue, Franklin Park, Illinois 60131.

CHAPTER 9

Vitamin E for Burns, Wounds, Bed Sores and Scars

"CAN ANYONE IMAGINE the total volume of pain, disability and scarring that follows burns?" asked Dr. Evan Shute in an address before the International Academy of Preventive Medicine. "Can anyone imagine the expense of hospital beds and physiotherapeutic pools, the loss of work and time, the deformities, amputations and such associated with burns and cuts?

"Extend this estimate over the centuries of recorded time. Remember that every living person is burned scores of times during his life and is often cut, often has wounds resisting the most versatile healing effects. Estimate the sum of pain alone and the prospect becomes literally overpowering," Dr. Shute went on.

Yet, he says, most of these problems are handled by "folk medicine" or remedies from the corner drug store. Doctors know next to nothing about treating wounds and burns. There is doubt among physicians, for example, as to whether wounds and burns should be covered with a dressing or if it's better to leave them open to the air. Considering the fact that such dreadful and disabling accidents have beset the human race since it appeared on this planet, it is shameful that medical science has no more effective treatment than it has produced up to now.

Dr. Shute tells us that he described the value of vitamin E for burns at the Second World Symposium on Vitamin E in 1949. So for 29 years the medical profession has known that such a therapy exists and has, in general, ignored it. One of the objections of the medical establishment to Dr. Shute's descriptions of burn treatment with vitamin E is that he has not used "controls." That is, he has not managed to observe two burned patients, one of which is treated with vitamin E, the other with traditional therapy, to decide which therapy is better.

Dr. Shute hoots with derision at the very idea of "controls" in burn treatment. He says, "No burn is or can be of the same depth as others, or involve the same surface area or vascular supply as any other." His treatment of burn patients with vitamin E, then, is "only anectodal." In other words, he has only the stories themselves, or the photographs of cured patients. "Of course," he says, "anectodal like digitalis and tolbutamide and plaster casts and coronary bypasses or heart transplants. Patients spend $3,000 to $6,000 on some of these items."

No, he says, he will not use controls for burn studies. And he proceeds to give us some "anecdotes" about patients he has treated with vitamin E. They are most convincing. Listen.

A six-year-old boy who, nine weeks before, had spilled scalding water over his back and chest. Skin grafts had not taken. When he was brought to Dr. Shute, he was covered with pus and "one could smell him six feet away." Dr. Shute treated him for 13 weeks before he was completely healed. **He was given 300 I.U. of vitamin E daily and vitamin E ointment was applied locally. No other treatment was used except for antibiotics on the septic wounds. He healed completely with no contracted scars.**

Another six-year-old boy dropped a hot iron on the

119

back of his hand, creating a second-degree burn. He was given 300 units of vitamin E daily, a sulfa ointment was applied to the burn for eight days, then vitamin E ointment. **In 31 days the hand was perfectly healed and all fingers could be flexed perfectly.** "Here is one of the most dramatic effects of alpha tocopherol (vitamin E)," says Dr. Shute. "It produces scars which do not contract as they heal."

A steelworker had dropped hot slag on his foot 11 months before he came to Dr. Shute. He had a dermatitis which would not heal. **He was given 400 units of vitamin E and ointment was applied locally. The foot and the dermatitis healed in 13 days.**

A 38-year-old man suffered second-degree burns in a gas explosion. He was severely blistered and skin was denuded over three fingers and the thumb. **On 300 units of vitamin E and vitamin E ointment he was completely healed in 11 days without the slightest impairment of flexion.**

A 14-year-old boy, run over by a truck 17 months before, had had skin grafts which had not taken, nor had the wound healed from which the grafted skin was taken. The boy was totally discouraged, emaciated, hopeless and had gone home to die. The grafts were covered with purulent scabs. He had bedsores from lying in one position. Dr. Shute treated the scabs with antibiotics, gave the boy 400 units of vitamin E daily, applied vitamin E ointment to the wounds and a vitamin E spray over them. **In two years the boy was completely well and able to engage in strenuous sports.** Now grown, he has only a slight limp.

A 53-year-old diabetic had a perforating ulcer on his foot, which was also dark purple, the color of a gangrenous foot. **On 375 units of vitamin E, he healed completely in 71 days.** And within several months his insulin requirement had decreased to about one-third of what it had been. He returned to work.

A five-year-old boy had developed keloid scars as a result of skin grafting for a bad burn. The scars were so itchy that the boy could not sit still in school and could not concentrate. **He was given vitamin E ointment only—none orally—and within days the itching disappeared and the boy became comfortable.**

A 24-year-old man was treated for severe burns by a professor of surgery, a famous plastic surgeon and a second surgeon. They published a joint paper in a medical journal on the great success they had treating this man. What they did not know, says Dr. Shute, was that the patient was a firm believer in vitamin E and had used the ointment himself throughout his treatment without mentioning it to the doctors.

A 46-year-old woman was burned severely on the right hand and arm. She was another believer in vitamin E. She took large doses of the vitamin by mouth, bandaged her arm and headed for the Shute Clinic. They treated her with saline bubble baths and vitamin E ointment. **In eight days she was almost completely recovered.** Dr. Shute states that he has colored photographs or X-ray pictures of all these cases. Yet vitamin E is almost unknown in the medical profession as a treatment for burns.

In the Foreword to *Vitamin E, Wonder Worker of the '70's?* by Ruth Adams and Frank Murray, Dr. Shute said, "Somehow and soon, I hope, doctors everywhere will feel free to use it (vitamin E), especially on burns. It hurts me to think that I described its use for burns as long ago as 1949... and that tocopherol still would not be tried if Hiroshima were repeated in Cairo or Jerusalem tomorrow. What misery and grafting and expense and hospital beds could have been saved had it been used in Nagasaki or were it even widely used now. I prefer not to think of such things. It lessens my esteem for my medical brethren and of mankind generally to think about all this.

"I suppose this guerilla warfare will continue, but some day soon... American medical authorities will concede to the irresistible firepower of vitamin E, leaving American doctors free to use it. How lucky we have been to live in Canada! I know how long we would have lasted in territory controlled by the American Medical Association. How many valuable ideas in medicine must have died aborting because its authorities made the going too heavy and young men simply gave up...."

One of the most stunning and dramatic stories is the story of the miracles wrought by vitamin E in treating stubborn ulcers and gangrene which had resisted all medical efforts at cure.

The treatment took place in a small-town hospital in Pennsylvania. It is reported by the nurse in charge and appears in *The Summary* for December, 1974. The publication is edited by Dr. Evan Shute.

One case is that of a 59-year-old woman with ulceration of the right foot. A diabetic, she was taking no medication when she came to the hospital. The doctors immediately gave her insulin and 800 units of natural vitamin E daily. Then they packed the ulcerated area with cotton saturated in vitamin E. Two months later all wounds were healed.

The second case is that of a 72-year-old woman with partial bowel obstruction and a huge bed sore (decubitus ulcer the doctors call it), which covered most of the upper part of her buttocks. A color photograph reveals a hideous festering sore with blackened areas. The ulcer was treated with daily applications of vitamin E and the patient was given 800 units of vitamin E by mouth every day. Treatment was begun on February 15, 1974 and was completed on August 12, 1974. Says Dorothy Fisher, who wrote this article, "In less than six months there was total healing and the area involved has remained well healed. The area now looks very healthy."

The third case is a 25-year-old man, a paraplegic, crippled in a car accident. Bedfast, he had developed bed sores on the buttocks, in the right leg and left foot. He had been treated without success in five different hospitals and rehabilitation institutions. He was given 400 units of vitamin E daily, plus 250 milligrams of vitamin C and his bed sores were treated topically with vitamin E ointment.

One month later his vitamin E and vitamin C dosages were doubled. A month later the vitamin E was increased to 600 units twice daily, later to 800 units twice daily.

He was sent home completely healed and is still taking 400 units of vitamin E daily, along with applications of the ointment to any area threatened with pressure sores.

The fourth case treated by this devoted nurse was a woman of 63 who was operated on for cancer of the rectum. The surgeon performed a colostomy. The opening or stoma which he created for evacuation of the bowel became infected and ulcerated. It and the area around it were treated daily with vitamin E ointment. The patient was given 400 units of vitamin E daily. **Within six days all this area of badly** ulcerated skin was completely healed.

Color photographs of these cases are printed with the article. It seems almost impossible to believe that any physician, aware of the benefits of vitamin E treatment, would not use it. It also seems incredible that official medicine has never published in any of its journals any material on using vitamin E in this way.

CHAPTER 10

Other Skin Disorders

A CALIFORNIA PHYSICIAN believes that vitamin E is so promising for treating a variety of skin disorders that double-blind studies should be done at once. Dr. Rees B. Rees of the University of California said that vitamin E has been tried with varying amounts of success in the following conditions: epidermolysis bullosa, Raynaud's phenomenon, scleroderma, calcinosis cutis, yellow nail syndrome, skin disorders associated with lupus erythematosus, as well as granuloma annulare, lichen sclerosis et atrophicus, porphyria cutanea tarda, pseudoxantome elasticum, subcorneal pustular dermatosis, necrobiosis lipoidica diabeticorum, Darier's disease, pityriasis rubra pilaris, cutaneous vasculitis, benign chronic familial pemphigus and chronic ulers. Some of these skin conditions have been treated by the Shute brothers of Canada, foremost champions of vitamin E for many ailments. Dr. Rees made his suggestion at a meeting of the American Academy of Dermatology. The meeting was reported in the February, 1974 issue of *Skin and Allergy News*.

A disease called dermolytic bullous dermatosis is one of the most disabling and heart-breaking. It is a skin disorder in which the patient is covered with blisters. To apply and change dressings sometimes requires half a day or more. Skin is so sensitive that some patients cannot endure the touch of anything on the surface of the skin. The blisters break and "weep" continually.

Two New Mexico physicians report on using vitamin E in the treatment of this disease. Writing in *Archives of Dermatology* for August, 1973 they tell us of two sisters who suffered from this excruciating disease. One of the sisters was given a drug which is used to treat this disease, the other was given vitamin E. **The vitamin E treatment caused a marked reduction in the formation of blisters while the drug had no such effect.**

Then the treatment was reversed and the sister who had gotten the vitamin E was given the drug, while the other sister got the vitamin E. Once again the vitamin gave immediate improvement while the drug achieved nothing. The mechanism of the action of vitamin E in this disease is unknown, say the authors, Dr. E. B. Smith and W. M. Michener of the University of New Mexico School of Medicine in Albuquerque.

In 1961, a 14-year-old boy was brought to a Canadian hospital from a home for incurable children where he had been for six years. The child was born with the blister disease. Approximately 10 hours of nursing care a day were required to care for him, including a half-hour bath twice daily, before the bandages on his arms and legs were removed.

Dr. H. D. Wilson, writing of this case in the *Canadian Medical Journal* for June 6, 1964 states: "The condition of his skin, when the dressings were removed, can scarcely be described. It is difficult to imagine a more unpleasant sight, compounded of blisters of all sizes, scabs, scars and bloody purulent discharge." The unfortunate child had suffered with this condition for 14 years. From head to foot he was one mass of fiery red ulceration. His mouth and throat were ulcerated, and so painful that he could eat only puréed food.

125

Because of his success in treating chronic varicose ulcers with vitamin E, Dr. Wilson decided to try this vitamin, although he could not discover in medical literature any case of such a patient being treated with the vitamin. He says, "The general appearance of the patient's face suggested vitamin deficiency, in spite of the multi-vitamins he had long been receiving."

There is no need to recount in detail the treatment given the boy. But all medication was stopped except vitamin E and a sedative. Four hundred units of vitamin E, four times a day was the initial dosage. This was soon increased to 800 units four times a day. The patient began to improve. His appetite increased. He gained weight. He became more cheerful. The blisters continued to appear but were smaller and more easily healed.

The dosage of vitamin E was increased to 1,200 units, four times a day and soon the sedative could be discontinued. The child improved so much that within eight months he could go for long outings in an automobile. Four months later, he was attending school; he was getting occupational therapy and his mental attitude had improved greatly.

The vitamin E was discontinued to see if the progress that had been made would continue. It did not. The boy's skin became worse again. So vitamin E was begun again and the dosage was increased to 6,000 units. **By the end of November, 1963, the skin condition was greatly improved and his knees and feet were nearly normal.**

Then, says Dr. Wilson, "the patient's mental attitude had improved, from one of depression, hopelessness and fault-finding to one characterized by better cooperation, more interest in his environment, and planning for the future. This change in mental outlook may be of some interest in view of the...reports of Del Guidice of Argentina on the effect of (vitamin E) on psychotic and behavioral problems of more advanced types." Dr. Wilson is speaking here of a physician who has reported promising results in treating mentally deficient and emotionally disturbed children with large doses of vitamin E.

The disease treated by Dr. Wilson is fortunately rare. The significant part of the story, it seems to us, is that he dared to discontinue all medication and use a plain vitamin in massive doses because he knew of its effectiveness in curing other kinds of ulcers. **It is interesting, too, that vitamin E can be taken in such large doses without any fear of the harmful side effects which most drugs produce.**

Then, too, we think this story indicates that there may be many disorders and conditions with which people are born, which may be related simply to lack of certain vitamins, or a need for some vitamin far greater than the average requirement. Isn't it possible that this child's difficulty was simply that he needed many thousands of times more vitamin E than the rest of us need?

As soon as the vitamin E was supplied in ample quantity, as much as he could possibly use, he began to improve. Perhaps there are many other conditions which will finally turn out to be caused simply by lack of one or more of the vitamins which this individual happens to need in enormous amounts.

The Summary for December, 1974, describes a number of cases of **epidermis bullosa**. Three cases in three generations of one family were treated with 300 milligrams of vitamin E daily with excellent results.

Another case involved two children, a seven-year-old girl and an eight-year-old boy, with epidermis bullosa acquista. **They were treated with vitamin E and improved to such an extent that the little girl could run and skip rope; the boy could play football.** The doctors began with doses of 200 units a day and recommended that, for severe eruptions, dosage as high as 800 to 1,600 units should be used. It is noteworthy that the disease improved only as long as the vitamin was given.

Purpura means hemorrhages in the skin, mucus membranes and other parts of the body. An article from the

127

Journal of Vitaminology, Vol. 18, page 125, 172, published in Japan, tells of seven cases of purpura treated with vitamin E. Four hundred to 600 milligrams of the vitamin were given daily and there was "marked clinical improvement." Six out of the seven cases improved with Vitamin E therapy alone.

It is interesting to note that, at the same time, the vitamin improved other conditions as well, such as local swelling (edema) and skin eruptions. **The authors believe this demonstrates that vitamin E prevents damage to capillary walls (the walls of the smallest blood vessels) when this damage is due to drugs, infections and so on.**

Systemic lupus erythematosus is a disorder which is most frequent in young women. It has a wide variety of symptoms involving many parts of the body. The skin is affected with ulcerating, blistering lesions. Heart, circulatory system and kidneys are affected. Painful arthritis is a common symptom. Pneumonia and pleurisy may be complications. The spleen may be affected. No one knows what causes the disorder, but apparently it can be triggered by a bad case of sunburn. Some patients must forever stay out of the sunlight, as it makes symptoms much worse.

A great deal of useful nutritional information is published in a quarterly newsletter, *Lupus Lifeline*. It is edited by Mrs. Betty Hull, Leanon (for L. E. Anonymous), P. O. Box 10243, Corpus Christi, Texas 78410.

Mrs. Hull, a plucky housewife, was stricken with this disorder over eight years ago. Cortisone and other drugs prescribed by her doctor to alleviate the condition only made matters worse. Her health began to improve when she started drinking large quantities of fresh carrot juice. This led to her interest in nutrition. Her health continued to improve as she began avoiding sugar, white flour and all processed foods. The disease has now been "in remission" for over eight years.

Mrs. Hull still drinks a cup of freshly juiced carrot juice each day. In addition, she takes the following supplements:

30,000 I.U. of vitamin A; B Complex vitamins (one or two a day depending on stress); Para-amino-benzoic-acid (PABA), the B vitamin that helps to screen out the sun's harmful rays, 100 milligrams; pantothenic acid, another B vitamin, 250 milligrams daily; niacin (vitamin B3), 100 milligrams daily; pyridoxine (vitamin B6), 50 milligrams twice daily; choline, another B vitamin, 250 milligrams daily; vitamin C, 3,000 milligrams daily; vitamin D, 2,500 milligrams daily; vitamin E, 1,000 milligrams daily. She began with very low doses of vitamin E because of high blood pressure, and increased them gradually up to her present daily intake.

As for minerals, Mrs. Hull takes the following: 6 bone meal tablets daily, 6 dolomite tablets daily, two to four kelp tablets daily, and a multi-mineral tablet. Apparently it was the calcium, phosphorus and magnesium plus the trace minerals in these fine mineral supplements which brought about the improvement in the spine condition which Mrs. Hull had thought would make her an invalid for life. The cortisone treatments, given for three years, had brought about demineralization of her spine.

"I believe in all this so strongly that I have yet to see anyone, with any disease, try this all the way and not be improved," says Mrs. Hull. She adds, "If you've tried nutrition/diet and it has helped you and your doctor notices it at check-up, let him know. Let's not keep this wonderful information hidden."

Lupus patients have difficulty with infections. Mrs. Hull manages them by increasing her intake of vitamin C every hour until she feels better.

There is no way of knowing whether these are exactly the food supplements you may happen to need, whether or not you suffer from lupus. Every individual is different, with differing requirements for nutrients. If you or some member of your family suffers from lupus, we urge you to write to Mrs. Hull and join her organization.

CHAPTER 11

Varicose Veins

IN THE BOOK, *Vitamin E for Ailing and Healthy Hearts*, by Dr. Wilfrid E. Shute and Harald Taub, a chapter on varicose veins relates astonishing stores of improvement of this unsightly, painful condition when vitamin E was given for other heart and circulatory conditions. The vitamin was given in massive doses. The doctor who gave it was the co-author, Dr. Shute.

He gives case histories of women who have had varicose veins for 50 years, aggravated by numerous pregnancies. **The veins have improved from the point of view of circulation and have decreased in size, when vitamin E was given in large doses.** Other patients had varicose veins along with phlebitis, eczema and swelling in the legs. Improvement was rapid with vitamin E.

Now consider the report of Dr. Harold Dodd, a British doctor, who stated in *The Lancet*, October 10, 1964 that varicose veins are all but unknown in certain people who eat differently from the way we Westerners eat.

Dr. Dodd made a survey in an African hospital in Zululand and found that, out of a total of 11,462 hospital patients (including maternity patients) and a total of 103,857 outpatients, there were only three women with varicose veins, one with hemorrhoids and several with other similar disorders. In England, an estimated 10 per cent of the total population suffers from varicose veins. Why should there be such a great difference between the two regions in the incidence of varicose veins?

Using evidence published by another British physician, Dr. T. L. Cleave, Dr. Dodd advances the theory that varicose veins are the direct result of a diet in which processed foods play a large part. Dr. Cleave believes that varicose veins are caused by a certain position of the colon which, when constipated, drags on one of the important large veins which return blood from the legs. As this condition goes on, year after year, it becomes increasingly difficult for blood to return to the heart from the legs, the valves in those veins begin to function badly and eventually varicose veins result.

Dr. Dodd checked on 100 patients in a British hospital with varicose vein troubles in their legs and found that "in two-thirds to three-fourths there was clear evidence of bowel irregularity." Many patients stated that they took laxatives regularly every day; others admitted that they resorted to laxatives when they missed a day's evacuation. A number of the patients had had trouble with hemorrhoids; others had had operations because of bowel difficulties.

In a later issue of *The Lancet*, Dr. Dodd's theory is challenged by another doctor, who claims that primitive Africans may not be subject to varicose veins because they walk much of the day, rather than riding or sitting. When they sit, they squat on the ground. He says that in Western countries obesity is a very prevalent condition from which these Africans do not suffer. This may have something to do with varicose veins. In addition, he says, obesity makes physical activity more difficult, so that walking and other exercises are shunned.

Dr. Dodd replies that varicose veins are quite prevalent among Western men who spend most of their day walking or working at hard manual labor but who eat the refined, processed diet of the Western world which is a certain cause of constipation because all the fibrous parts of the cereals have been removed.

Dr. Cleave, who originated the idea that varicose veins are another by-product of our modern diet, has told us in other publications that heart disease, tooth decay and peptic ulcer are also by-products of our modern diet. Dr. Cleave is a proponent of a diet as completely natural as possible—that is, with as few changes as possible being made when the food is prepared. He says, furthermore, that one should eat whatever he wishes, and should eat only foods for which he is hungry. Provided he sticks to wholly natural foods that have not been denatured in any way, he cannot possibly suffer any harm from such a diet, but will instead find his health improving every day.

What would such a diet consist of? Dr. Dodd calls it "The 1,000-year-old diet." It consists, he says, of "reasonable amounts of meat, fish, poultry, fresh eggs and cheese, wholemeal bread, fresh fruit, nuts, raisins, salads and vegetables. With the addition of one or two tablespoons of unprocessed bran daily, this diet has ensured for many Britons two smooth, effortless stools a day without need of aperients (laxatives)."

Note that such a diet omits completely the starchy and sugar laden foods which make up such a large part of the diet of most Americans. There are no cakes, pastry, doughnuts, pasta, candy, chewing gum, soft drinks, rolls or muffins, except for the completely whole grain kind. Dr. Cleave goes even farther, for he believes that all food should have as little preparation as possible. In other words, a fresh raw apple is better for you than applesauce, and if you are hungry for an apple, don't eat applesauce or apple pie. Eat an apple.

In a later issue of *The Lancet*, another physician praises the ideas of Drs. Dodd and Cleave, and adds his own comment on bran. Says he: "There can be no doubt about the value of unprocessed bran in the management of constipation. In general practice I have found unprocessed

132

bran particularly beneficial in the elderly and in pregnancy. Recently a patient in early pregnancy, so constipated that she was able to empty her bowels only by weekly enemas, achieved natural movement and relief from symptoms of nausea and pain by the use of bran.

"Unprocessed bran is cheap," he goes on, "and in action has none of the gripeing or excessive purgation effects which can be so distressing when bowel stimulants are used. I am sure that it is a healthier remedy than the various combinations of liquid paraffin (mineral oil).

"May I record my hearty agreement with Dr. Dodd's plea for a reform of our eating habits and with his view that the benefits of unprocessed foods should be publicized."

In the December 9, 1972 issue of *The Lancet*, Dr. Cleave says, "Since varicose veins are so common in our population who eat a mass of refined carbohydrate and have a prolonged transit-time but are almost unknown in those populations subsisting on unrefined carbohydrates and having a halved transit-time in consequence, is it not vital at least to consider the removal of a colonic-pressure cause on the external iliac veins at the pelvic brim? . . . The halving of the intestinal transit-time (that is, the relief of constipation) can be secured very easily by the taking of unprocessed bran at the cost of only a few pence a month and is in full swing in at least one British hospital. . . . With over 5 million cases of varicose veins in this country and over 7 million people on habitual purgatives, there is room for this study."

A letter to the editor of the *Journal of the American Medical Association* asks what is recommended for a 12-year-old boy whose entire family is afflicted with varicose veins. The boy is already a victim and has had several operations. The expert who replies recommends that overweight should be avoided. All family members should avoid long periods of standing or sitting with their feet hanging down. They should never cross their legs. They should engage in vigorous exercises like bicycling, walking

133

and swimming. They should avoid any tight clothing like garters or girdles. Any member of the family with varicose veins should wear elastic stockings and should sleep with the foot of the bed elevated three or four inches, he said.

An American foot doctor reports in the *Journal of the American Podiatry Association* on 72 patients who complained of foot and leg problems: cold feet and legs, night cramps, chronic phlebitis, varicose ulcers, diabetic ulcers, tired feet and legs. **Sixty-five of them showed improvement with 600 units of vitamin E daily, reduced gradually**. Improvement began in about six weeks.

In a booklet, *Common Questions on Vitamin E and Their Answers*, by the staff of the Shute Foundation for Medical Research, London, Ontario, Canada, the question is asked: "Is vitamin E used to treat varicose veins?" The reply follows:

"We originally refused to treat such patients, thinking it was absurd to believe that vitamin E had anything to offer them. But so many patients with such leg conditions, whom we treated for other cardiovascular (heart) diseases, told us how much their varices (varicose veins) improved that we finally decided it was worthy of trial, and now we have become thoroughly convinced of its value."

As a result of the Shute's experiences with vitamin E in treating varicose veins, they came to the conclusion, they say, that everyone with varicose veins should try vitamin E before even considering an operation. They have found, they say, that operations may have very poor results.

CHAPTER 12

Buerger's Disease

A CHRONIC DISEASE of the arteries and veins, Buerger's Disease usually affects the extremities. But it can involve any blood vessels of the body. It is also known as Thrombo-angiitis Obliterans.

With this disease, a gradual thrombosis or narrowing of the blood vessel eventually interferes with the blood supply to the affected part and gangrene results, according to *Medigraph Manual*, by Dr. George E. Paley and Herbert C. Rosenthal.

"The disease is thought to be hereditary," the medical encyclopedia continues. "Patients are almost always men, and most have a history of heavy smoking. Another unexplained fact about Buerger's disease is that 50 per cent of the victims are of Jewish parentage."

According to *Medigraph Manual*, the first symptom is usually a crampy pain in the calves or arches brought on by walking or running. As the disease progresses, it takes less and less activity to produce pain, which eventually becomes constant.

"Phlebitis—inflammation in which the veins become swollen, red and painful to touch—is usually associated with Buerger's," the book continues. "The nails become brittle and grow slowly, and there is ulceration of the toes. Color changes take place. In the beginning the extremity is

135

usually cold to touch and pale in color. Later on, depending upon where the disease is established, the affected part may be deep red or blue—depending on its position. When it is elevated, it may turn white; when it is hanging down, it becomes dark. As time passes there is a tendency for the skin to infect easily. There are ulcerations. Eventually gangrene may develop, accompanied by severe, persistent pain... There have been some reports of coronary or cerebral artery involvements resulting in stroke or coronary attacks."

Buerger's Disease may begin in men who are quite young, especially smokers. Tobacco has been incriminated as the chief cause of this circulatory disorder. **Vitamin E in large amounts appears to give prompt relief which is extraordinary since no other therapy appears to accomplish anything.** Along with vitamin E, it is, of course, absolutely necessary to stop smoking. Not just cut down, but stop.

In a Hungarian medical journal, Dr. F. Gerloczy tells of the beneficial effects of vitamin E on a number of people suffering from various circulatory disorders. He gave the vitamin in enormous doses—up to 24,000 milligrams or units daily. **In some diseases, "spectacular" results were obtained:** in 10 cases of thrombosis of the arteries, 16 cases of thrombophlebitis, and 12 out of 15 cases of Buerger's Disease. In other cases of circulatory troubles, the doctor reported great relief in some patients, little improvement in others. One patient who had had a leg ulcer for 20 years was healed completely after only six weeks on vitamin therapy internally, plus vitamin E ointment on the skin.

In the December, 1972 issue of *The Summary*, Dr. Evan Shute, the editor, says that Buerger's Disease is the sinister and usually hopeless condition in which circulation in legs becomes so bad that recovery is impossible and amputation is needed. **"Vitamin E saves many such legs,"** Dr. Shute says. And he reports that there are 13 papers in medical literature attesting to this fact.

136

CHAPTER 13

Vitamin E for Gum Health

IN THE July 8, 1972 issue of *Science News*, it was announced that a University of California dental researcher has found that vitamin E is apparently valuable in the treatment of gum disease or pyorrhea. There is some evidence, says Dr. J. Max Goodson, that bacteria may create substances called prostaglandins, along with inflammation in the gums. This researcher is working to find something that will counteract the prostaglandins.

Vitamin E seems to work. The California scientist experimented with 16 patients with gum disease. He gave them 800 milligrams of vitamin E each day for 21 days. At the same time he gave a capsule containing nothing at all to 10 other patients with pyorrhea.

Then he measured the amount of inflammation as evidenced by the fluid around the patients' teeth in each group. **It appeared that there had been a significant decrease in the fluid around the teeth of those who got the vitamin E supplement.** The other patients' teeth remained the same.

Dr. Goodson reminds us that it's possible that reversing the inflammatory process in the gums may not wipe out the disease. But the two conditions always go hand in hand. He plans to investigate still other substances which also inhibit prostaglandins. Meanwhile, there is no reason why the rest of us cannot use the information he has published for our own benefit. In case you've been taking vitamin E and have noticed improvement in the condition of your gums, it seems quite possible that the vitamin E was at least partly responsible.

Dental Abstracts for September, 1973 tells of 14 patients with gum (periodontal) disease. They were given 800 milligrams of vitamin E daily. **The vitamin reduced inflammation after 21 days, so it should help to prevent bone loss in the jaw.**

In *Proceedings of the Workshop on Diet, Nutrition and Periodontal Disease*, the just-named Dr. J. Max Goodson is worried about the amount of unsaturated fats which Americans are eating these days, and the amount of vitamin E that may be necessary because of this intake of PUFA—or polyunsaturated fatty acids as they are called.

Dr. Goodson tells us that 40 per cent of the American diet is fat and about 17 per cent of this is unsaturated fat. So the average diet contains about 17 grams of PUFA. According to the recommended ratio of PUFA to vitamin E, the person eating this much PUFA should certainly have 10 milligrams of vitamin E in his meals. If corn oil is substituted for *all* other fats in the diet, 33 milligrams of vitamin E would be necessary as a minimum.

There is a present trend to increase intake of PUFA, mostly because it is believed to reduce the amount of cholesterol in the blood. The impact of this trend means that we should all be certain we are getting enough vitamin E. If we are concentrating on getting lots of PUFA in margarine, salad oils, and so on, then we must be extra careful to get enough vitamin E.

Dr. Goodson goes on to say that the quantity of vitamin E in food is depleted by processing. Whole wheat bread contains four times more vitamin E than white bread. Most of us eat white bread. Ordinary cooking does not destroy much of the vitamin E in food, but when foods that have been fried in vegetable oil are then frozen, thawed and eaten, most vitamin E is lost. This would apply to things like frozen French Fries and so on.

According to surveys done, says Dr. Goodson, **from 2 to 12 per cent of our population have blood levels of vitamin E which are less than 0.5 milligrams per cent. At this level of deficiency, red blood cells are destroyed.** One-third of us have blood levels of vitamin E below one milligram—the level required to completely eliminate this destruction of red blood cells.

This destruction would, presumably, be involved in causing bleeding gums. And, sure enough, a study has shown that there is considerable less bleeding in individuals with high blood levels of vitamin E. Other surveys have shown that getting more vitamin E and having higher blood levels as a result are associated with better gum health. And the opposite condition (too little vitamin E) is associated with poor health of the gums.

In animals, lack of vitamin E does not produce gum disease or pyorrhea as we call it, but it does result in thinner membranes in certain gum tissues. Giving rats 60 milligrams of vitamin E every other day (an enormous amount for an animal the size of a rat) arrested this destructive process but did not restore the gums to their original health.

Giving vitamin E to human beings has been effective in reducing signs of inflammation and in holding teeth more firmly in the gums. In patients with a muscle-wasting disease, 30 milligrams of vitamin E were given in intramuscular injections once or twice weekly. The condition of the gums of all such patients improved, usually by the fourth week. The color of the gums returned to normal. They stopped bleeding. The teeth which had been very loose before gradually became tighter in their sockets.

Another dentist quoted by Dr. Goodson reported

improvement in loose teeth—with no other treatment than vitamin E being given. It is well to remember that more teeth are lost to gum disorders, after middle age, than are lost to tooth decay. The volume of fluid in certain gum tissues has been found to correlate with the amount of pyorrhea present. Twenty-six patients were given 800 milligrams a day of vitamin E, which was rinsed about the mouth before swallowing so that it could come into contact with the gums. There was a significant decrease in the amount of fluid present, indicating that the gum condition had improved.

As reported in Dr. Goodson's earlier article, there are substances called prostaglandins which are manufactured from fatty acids when they are oxidized—that is, combined with oxygen. One of these has been incriminated as a cause of inflammation in gums and the destruction of the bones in which the teeth are fixed. In laboratory experiments, vitamin E prevents the formation of this harmful substance.

Dr. Goodson tells us that experiments have also shown that rats exposed to ozone and nitrogen dioxide (two urban air pollutants) live longer when their diets are supplemented with vitamin E. Says Dr. Goodson, "These studies suggest that the human dietary requirement for vitamin E may be further elevated by pollution of the environment with oxidant gases."

This ties in, also, with the bleeding gums that occur in gum disease. Lack of vitamin E makes the red blood cells especially susceptible to destruction when these oxidizing pollutants are present. If there is a generalized decrease in the ability of the gum cells to maintain their cell walls, the tissues will gradually be destroyed.

How much vitamin E should one take to guard against gum troubles? Dr. Goodson tells us that 60 milligrams a day should be enough to protect even that individual who is taking very large amounts of unsaturated fats. He tells us, too, that another researcher says that more than 500 milligrams a day do not produce an increase in the effectiveness of the vitamin in protecting us from various health problems.

But blood levels of more than one milligram are apparently necessary to protect from bleeding gums. And to get this high a level in the blood one would have to take at least 60 or more milligrams of vitamin E a day. "In contrast to the fat-soluble vitamins A and D," says Dr. Goodson, "vitamin E has no recognized toxicity. As much as 40,000 milligrams a day have been given with no observable ill effects."

He goes on to say that, "Considering the small number of controlled clinical experiments, some with serious deficiencies in design, one cannot conclude without reservation that vitamin E offers therapeutic benefit in the treatment of periodontal disease. However, this effect can be predicted from our knowledge of its biochemical action and has been reported by clinicians who have tested it."

What happens is that inflammation is improved and loose teeth become more firmly fixed in the gums. This is often without any accompanying treatment. At least 30 milligrams a day should be prescribed by the dentist or doctor treating the disease.

Get plenty of vitamin E in capsules, especially if you are taking unsaturated fats in margarine or salad oil or under a doctor's direction. Take plenty of vitamin E if you consistently eat white bread and processed cereals, for almost all of this vitamin has been removed from these foods which were originally, in their wholegrain state, our best sources of this vitamin.

If you ask the average dentist what are the causes of gingivitis and pyorrhea, he will probably tell you the conditions are due to particles of food stuck in pockets in the gums, close to teeth. These then become infected, so the story goes and the teeth sometimes loosen. Therapy is often quite expensive and time-consuming. Teeth are often lost.

Dr. E. Cheraskin of the University of Alabama,

Department of Oral Medicine, has been interested for many years in the effect of sugar and refined carbohydrates on various functions of the body. Among the many valuable papers he has authored along these lines is one which appeared in the *Journal of Oral Medicine* for April, 1966, in which Dr. Cheraskin and his associates describe an experiment involving 118 healthy dental students to discover what effect, if any, a high carbohydrate diet would have on the condition of their gums. Then, too, the scientists tested actual drinks high in two sugars—glucose and sucrose.

One group was asked to eat a diet high in protein, low in refined carbohydrates. Other groups were given two daily drinks of sucrose—that is, very high in sugar, and glucose, another kind of sugar. Still another group was given a low-calorie drink, prepared with artificial sweeteners.

The condition of the subjects' gums was evaluated before the tests began and at their close. The examination was based on four conditions: no gingivitis present at all, or slight swelling of the gums, or moderate swelling and redness, plus tendency to bleed, with possible tenderness and pain. The fourth category was one in which there was marked redness and swelling, loss of tissue tone, spontaneous bleeding, possible ulceration, tenderness and pain. The doctors who examined the students at the end of the experiment had no knowledge of what kind of diet or drinks any one of them had been taking, so there could be no chance of anyone making the results fit a preconceived notion.

Results of the test showed that the greatest reduction in gum troubles was found in the group which ate the high protein, low carbohydrate diet with no sugared drink at all. The students who ended up with the worst mouth conditions were those who had 225 grams of glucose daily, and those who had 100 grams of sucrose daily. Students who drank the low-calorie drink, with no sugar, had a decrease in mouth and gum symptoms. And those who made no changes at all in their diet showed no changes in mouth and gum conditions.

It is surprising, these authors think, that a test of only three or four days could show such results. They say in their summary that refined carbohydrates play an important part in gum troubles. They do not know how. "Surely," they say, "the addition and elimination of refined carbohydrates alters the entire endocrine pattern"—that is, the way the glands work. So the changes in gum health may be due to some change in hormones.

"Also," they say, "there is suggestive evidence that the vitamin and trace mineral state varies directly with carbohydrate metabolism. (That is, the amount of carbohydrate eaten regulates the amount of vitamins and trace minerals that should be eaten.) "There is, then," they go on, "the possibility that the gingival (gum) findings may be associated with the various vitamins and particularly the vitamin B complex as well as certain trace minerals. It is a clinical fact that the intake of carbohydrates and proteins is almost inversely related. In other words, the individual who consumes large amounts of carbohydrate foods frequently does not ingest much protein. Therefore, the possibility exists here that protein metabolism is modified when refined carbohydrate foodstuffs are added and subtracted."

We think this is an extremely important piece of research. It shows that the health of your gums can be influenced by only a few days of addiction to sweets, even though you customarily eat a good high protein diet. Its authors believe it may demonstrate that the inclusion of refined carbohydrates in a diet may affect the way all body glands function. The authors also make the important point that the more starchy and sweet foods you eat, the less you will be inclined to eat of protein foods.

If a few days' exposure to a lot of sugar can do this to gums, think what damage can be done over a lifetime! Note, too, that low-calorie drinks did not produce gum damage. On the contrary, they appeared to lessen it. We suppose this may be because students who had low calorie drinks did not drink the usual sugar-sweetened soft drinks they customarily drank when they were not being tested.

We know well—and all dentists and dental researchers know well—just how much damage is done to teeth by sugar. When sugar is kept in constant contact with teeth over long periods of time, as when sticky candy is eaten or gum is chewed, teeth are destroyed wholesale. Now there seems to be ample evidence that sugar does just about as much damage to gums.

We say sugar because the starch of refined carbohydrates is changed to sugar. And if the effect on gums is something which is brought about by the sugar's effect on glands—and Dr. Cheraskin believes that it is—then this is an urgent reason for cutting down sharply on all refined carbohydrates. This means all foods that are mostly white flour or refined cereals or sugar, or anything made chiefly of these.

What should you substitute, if you are hoping for excellent gum health? Substitute foods high in protein, which are also those that contain most vitamins and minerals: meats, poultry, fish, eggs, cheese, milk and those vegetable foods highest in protein, like real whole cereals, beans and peas, seeds of all kinds, and nuts. Plus, of course, all those fresh fruits and vegetables which bring such good health benefits.

Dr. Cheraskin and two of his colleagues have also written what is probably the most valuable book available anywhere on the subject of diet in relation to gum and mouth disorders. Unfortunately it is too technical for the average layman. It was written for dentists. It is full of information on diet and its relation to the condition of all the mouth tissues.

Many experiments are described like the ones we mention in this chapter, involving many more people. In every case poor nutrition and poor eating habits brought

144

disaster. Good diet and plenty of vitamins and minerals brought improvement.

We earnestly recommend that you tell your doctor and your dentist about this book, if they do not already know of it. It is *Diet and the Periodontal Patient*, by Drs. James W. Clark, E. Cheraskin and W. M. Ringsdorf, Jr. It is published by Charles C. Thomas, Springfield, Illinois.

For health-seekers who are not professional scientists, Drs. Cheraskin and Ringsdorf have written an extremely helpful book on nutrition and health, *New Hope for Incurable Diseases*. You can probably find a copy at your health food store.

CHAPTER 14

Vitamin E
and Selenium
Are Related

"THE STEPCHILD OF SULFUR" is what Dr. Carl Pfeiffer calls the trace mineral selenium in his book, *Mental and Elemental Nutrients*. He adds that it is one of the most poisonous elements in the universe, and yet it has been found to be essential to life in animals and human beings.

This is not a mineral which you can slather all over your breakfast cereal and feel fine as a result. It is measured in foods and in soil in parts per million or in parts per billion. These are very small amounts indeed. Dr. Pfeiffer suggests that an adequate intake for human beings is probably about the same as that for animals—about 200 parts per billion.

Because just a bit too much selenium can be highly toxic and just a bit too little can cause disease, scientists have been busy investigating just what this trace mineral does in the body and how it does it. They have found that it is an essential part of at least two enzymes. Enzymes are chemical substances in cells which cause certain reactions to take place which could not take place without them. In one of these enzymes, glutathione peroxidase, selenium is the only trace mineral that can be found. So there is just no possibility of that enzyme performing as it should unless there is just a bit of selenium present to take part in the process.

Unless, of course, there is plenty of vitamin E around. For some reason, which nobody has quite untangled as yet, **selenium and vitamin E work closely together and sometimes one of them can substitute for the other.** So somebody faced with terrible deficiency in selenium in his food and water may get along considerably better if he has enough vitamin E. And vice versa.

It seems rather unlikely that such a circumstance would occur, however, since the germ and bran of cereals like wheat, which are the best sources of both selenium and vitamin E, are removed during the refining process. The white flour and processed cereals that result are therefore deficient in both the trace mineral and the vitamin, as well as many other minerals and vitamins.

It was only when stock animals began to get just a bit too much selenium in their fodder that animal scientists became concerned about this substance. Eating grass or grain raised on soil too rich in selenium can have serious health consequences for animals. On the other hand, getting too little selenium can apparently be very serious for human beings or animals. This can happen if one lives in a part of the country where there is too little selenium in soil and water. Or it can happen if one avoids those foods which contain reasonably adequate amounts of selenium, or if one devotes most of mealtime to eating foods grown on soil deficient in selenium or foods from which all selenium has been removed.

At a recent symposium of the International Association of Bioinorganic Scientists, several exciting prospects were suggested relative to preventing some of our most serious health calamities by getting enough selenium.

For instance, Dr. Gerhard Schrauzer of the University of California has studied a group of laboratory mice who have been bred for many generations to be highly susceptible to breast cancer. During their two-year lifespan, 80 to 100 per cent of these mice normally develop breast cancer.

Dr. Schrauzer and his colleagues gave the mice in their food 2 parts per million of a form of selenium. Over the lifetime of the mice only 2 per cent of the animals got breast cancer. In other words, only two out of every 100 of these mice developed the disease, although 80 to 100 out of every 100 mice would normally have developed breast cancer without the selenium supplement.

Incidence of **breast cancer** is rapidly rising among women in our country, although it is rare in certain other countries.

Dr. Schrauzer studied the levels of selenium in the blood of people from 17 countries and compared this with the number of cancer deaths in each country. **He found that in those countries where people had more selenium in their blood, there were fewer deaths from cancer.**

What about breast cancer? In Japan and other countries where the average levels of selenium in blood ranged from 0.26 parts per million to 0.29 parts per million, the breast cancer rate was from 0.8 to 8.5 per 100,000 population. In the United States and other Western countries where the level of blood selenium is lower—ranging from 0.07 to 0.20 parts per million, the breast cancer rate is much higher— 16.9 to 23.3 cases per 100,000 population.

If we want to lower the breast cancer rate in this country, says Dr. Schrauzer, we should try to shift the emphasis of our diet so that we get as much selenium as people in general do in the Far Eastern countries where breast cancer is much less prevalent. This means cutting way back on our consumption of sugar. We should reduce this to one-tenth of its present level, says Dr. Schrauzer. We should eat more wholegrain cereals and fish, both rich in selenium.

One of the reasons why selenium may be a powerful preventive of cancer is that it is an essential part of an important enzyme system, as we mentioned earlier. This enzyme system (the glutathione peroxidase system) is involved in preventing the unsaturated fats in our cells from oxidizing or becoming rancid. Another role of selenium in our bodies is to operate in a group of compounds called the sulfydryl group, which is active in many enzyme systems. One of their functions involves the process of cell division. Cancer is a disease in which cells divide wildly and erratically. Perhaps an unbalance of the restraining enzyme systems, caused by lack of selenium, may be one reason for the onset of cancer.

Still another function of selenium, Dr. Schrauzer believes, is to help the body's immune defense mechanism. This is the elaborate machinery the body puts into motion when its cells are threatened by invaders of many kinds, such as viruses and bacteria. Cancer cells are also invaders which the body tries to protect itself against. Perhaps the selenium that is available in every cell helps in this process.

Another distinguished scientist who participated at the trace mineral symposium was Dr. Raymond Shamberger of the Cleveland Clinic. Dr. Shamberger has been feeding mice chemical compounds which are known to cause cancer in all animals to which they are given. He has been giving one group of mice these compounds and another group of matched animals the same risky chemicals, but adding just a tiny bit of selenium to their chow. The selenium apparently protected the mice, since they did not get the cancers which ravaged the other group of mice.

The Cleveland researchers have also experimented with human cells in testtubes along with chemicals known to cause cancer. Adding a small amount of selenium to half of the test tubes prevents the breakage of cell walls which leads to cancer, so these cells are protected.

Dr. Shamberger was the first selenium researcher to study soil and water for traces of this mineral. Several years ago he found, to his surprise, that in areas of our country where there is plenty of selenium in the soil and water there are fewer cases of cancer than in those communities where there is very little selenium in soil and water. City by city, the Cleveland biologist compared disease statistics in 34 cities and found that in 17 where there is little selenium in soil and water cancer incidence is much higher than in those cities where selenium is relatively plentiful.

Later, Dr. Shambeger and and a colleague, Dr. Charles E. Willis, compared records of circulatory disorders related to high blood pressure in states where soil is rich in selenium and states where there is much less selenium. **They found that people in the low-selenium states are three times more susceptible to these circulatory problems.**

The more healthy, selenium-rich states are: Texas, Oklahoma, Arizona, Colorado, Louisiana, Utah, Alabama, Nebraska and Kansas. The states where soil is low in selenium are: Connecticut, Illinois, Ohio, Oregon, Massachusetts, Rhode Island, New York, Pennsylvania, Indiana and Delaware. No one can say unequivocally that the presence or absence of selenium in soil and water is the only thing influencing the rate of circulatory diseases in these localities. But isn't it significant that careful studies of disease statistics of millions of people seem to show a relation between the amount of selenium available to them in food and water and the amount of both cancer and circulatory diseases to which they are susceptible?

The Food and Drug Administration now permits the addition of selenium in trace amounts to feeds for stock animals like hogs, cattle and poultry. But there is evidence that the selenium content of our soils may be decreasing, so that food eaten by human beings may contain less and less selenium as time goes on.

There is not much selenium in artificial fertilizers. This kind of fertilizer also makes it difficult for the roots of plants to absorb selenium from the soil. The selenium in animal manure seems to be not available for plant roots. And the small amount of selenium in the air, which is given off when coal is burned, is also not in a form that is available to plant roots.

And, as we stated previously, scientists have found a mysterious relationship between selenium and vitamin E. It seems they work together in many helpful body functions in which both are involved. Working with animals, researchers have found that if selenium is scarce in the diet, vitamin E may help to prevent any disease which may follow. If there is too little vitamin E, then the available selenium may take the place of the vitamin and help to prevent anticipated diseases. But scientists have also found that, even if an animal or a human being is getting plenty of vitamin E, there are still additional health benefits from getting enough selenium as well.

But isn't it possible, especially if you live in a selenium-rich area, that you are already getting enough of this trace mineral? Possibly, if you eat locally grown produce and avoid sugar and white flour products. But for people living in the selenium-poor areas, it would be necessary not only to avoid these mineral-poor foods, but also to be certain that their fresh produce and grains come from areas where there is plenty of selenium in the soil. There doesn't seem to be any way for most of us to find out where our foods come from unless we raise them ourselves. And unless they are organically grown it seems certain our foods would suffer from selenium deficiency since commercial fertilizers impoverish the soil, especially where selenium is concerned.

In *The Lancet* for March 1, 1975, Dr. Eldon W. Keinholz of Colorado State University relates his troubles with pain in his knees after strenuous leg work. "The condition became worse," he says, "until in 1973 I was almost unable to complete a hike in nearby mountains because of pain. The problem was identified by an orthopedic surgeon as ligament irritation on lateral and frontal parts of the knee joint. I was recommended to accept the situation since there was no accepted therapy.

"I learned that selenium ingestion has been suggested as

151

a method of relieving some types of arthritis. In January, 1974, I began to ingest gelatin capsules, each containing one milligram of sodium selenite plus 68 milligrams of d-alpha tocopherol succinate (vitamin E). One capsule was taken regularly with meals every third day. A week before a hike in September, 1974 I ran approximately one-half mile each day (as I had done before hikes in previous years) and I increased my selenium and vitamin E intake into one capsule per day. Insofar as I was able to plan the experiment, everything was the same as in previous years with the exception of my selenium and vitamin E intake. I hiked 11 miles in one day, ascending and descending 2,875 feet with absolutely no knee discomfort. This contrasted with past hikes, especially one . . . in which the distance was identical but I only ascended and descended 1,685 feet and knee pain was nearly unbearable during the last 20 per cent of the hike. . . .

"I hope that the success of this small personal experiment will encourage further research into vitamin E and/or selenium therapy of arthritis problems in human knee joints. However the hazards of selenium supplementation must be borne in mind—one milligram of selenium supplement per day probably approaches the adult human toxicity levels. The vitamin E levels did not exceed those in widespread use."

Dr. Milton L. Scott of Cornell University reported at a meeting of the American Societies for Experimental Biology that selenium, acting as part of an enzyme, destroys certain unhealthy byproducts of fatty substances in the blood. These substances are destructive of the walls of capillaries, the smallest of the blood vessels. **Selenium destroys the harmful substances after they have appeared.**

It now seems that one of the roles of vitamin E is to prevent these fatty substances from forming. So the vitamin and the trace mineral work together—the vitamin prevents the harmful substances from forming. If not enough of the vitamin is present to do the job, selenium takes over and destroys the fatty byproducts that have formed.

It all sounds terribly complex to a non-chemist, but it demonstrates clearly the great complexity of the things that go on inside our bodies. In this case, getting enough vitamin E gives protection. But if the diet lacks vitamin E, the selenium can be depended upon to stop the next step toward ill-health. If both are lacking in the diet, disaster may result.

It may be years until some researcher gets around to discovering whether this same mechanism operates in human beings, and still more years until we get an official recommendation that our diets include selenium—in small quantities—and vitamin E in large enough amounts to protect us.

The National Academy of Sciences, National Research Council, whose scientific consultants decide officially how much we need of vitamins and minerals, have said that a daily supplement of 50 to 100 micrograms of selenium could be taken safely if there is any doubt about the possible levels of selenium in the diet. A specialist in trace minerals from Cornell University, the just mentioned Dr. Scott, believes that the average American gets about 25 to 100 micrograms daily from air, water and food. And he thinks it would be safe for us to get as much as 1,100 micrograms a day. An expert from the Department of Agriculture thinks the average American may be getting about 98 to 225 micrograms daily.

Of course, the amount you get depends mostly on what foods you eat and do not eat. If most of your diet consists of refined carbohydrates, you are probably desperately in need of selenium, no matter what else you eat. Seafood and meat—especially organ meats like liver and kidney—are good sources of selenium. Really wholegrain cereals are likely to be good sources, depending on where the grains were raised. Eggs may be good sources, depending on the amount of selenium in the diet of the hens which laid them.

Brewers yeast, which you can get at your health food store, is an excellent source of selenium. There are also food supplements available containing selenium, many of them derived from yeast. The chemical form of the selenium in such a supplement makes it more easily absorbed by the body, hence more useful and economical.

Vegetarians, studiously avoiding both seafood and meat, should watch carefully their intake of cereals to make certain they are always wholegrain. If possible, they should find out where these grains were grown. They should use brewers yeast in cooking or in beverages as another source of selenium as well as B vitamins and many other minerals.

People whose families have a history of cancer-susceptibility, especially breast cancer, and perhaps circulatory disorders as well, should go out of their way to get enough selenium. People who live in areas where soil and water are low in selenium should take selenium supplements probably, if they grow their own food or buy mostly food that was locally grown. And what is most important, all of us should begin now, if we haven't already, to eliminate those most harmful and deficient foods which contribute no selenium and almost no other trace mineral nutriment—the refined carbohydrates like white bread and commercial cereals, as well as white sugar and every food that contains it.

CHAPTER 15

Natural vs. Synthetic Vitamin E

HAVE YOU OFTEN WONDERED what the difference is between synthetic and natural vitamin E? The following material is reprinted from information supplied by Eastman Chemical Products, a manufacturer of natural vitamin E. It should answer most of your questions.

Vitamin E was discovered in 1922 in the course of biochemical research with laboratory animals. Over the years, thousands of scientific papers have been published on the subject. Much research on it is still going on in well-respected laboratories around the world.

Despite this half century of research, much less is known about the extent of the biological role of vitamin E than of a number of other vitamins.

In research, the effects of a lack of a vitamin can be studied by controlling the diet fed to animals. However, vitamin E is unusual in the large variation of effects among animal species from insufficient vitamin E. For example, in male rats the lack of vitamin E results in sterility; in calves, heart failure; in lambs, paralysis of the hind quarters; in chicks, leakage from the capillaries and brain deterioration; and in milk cows, bad flavored milk.

Even deciding on the recommended daily allowance of vitamin E is complicated. It depends very much on what else the animal is getting. For example, in cat food switching from one kind of fish product to another resulted in greatly increased need for vitamin E. When these increased needs were not met, pets died. ...

To serve the human need to make one's own choices, the marketplace offers such things as dietary supplements in such forms as capsules, tablets and liquids. Some of these are represented as "natural" in origin in contrast with "synthetic." ...

The particular kind of molecule that gives vitamin E effects is a structure of carbon, hydrogen and oxygen atoms. Molecules composed of these atoms are called "organic" because of a belief among early chemists that a certain category of substances could come only from living organisms. Today, scientists know how to make millions of kinds of "organic" molecules that never occur in nature, in addition to other thousands that do occur in nature. A "synthetic" molecule may be absolutely identical in every known property with one made by the body of a plant or a creature other than a human chemist.

It *may* be. It may also be slightly different. The difference, if any, may not matter for some purposes. For others it may matter.

Look at a glove for the right hand and its mate for the left hand. Same design, same material, but different. Molecules made by nature can differ from otherwise identical ones made by the chemist in just this property of "handedness." Only certain molecular structures have handedness, just as some familiar objects like dishes, for example, have no inbuilt handedness, while gloves and screw threads do have it. Vitamin E molecules have it, too.

When factories make molecules, the processes have to be efficient. Efficient methods of quantity production leave it to chance whether the parts of each individual molecule will be assembled left-handed or right-handed where either twist is possible. Nature, using subtle methods, tends to put them together with all the same twist.

In the case of vitamin E, a difference in twist makes a difference in biological potency. This is officially recognized in National Formulary's definition of the International Unit of vitamin E, the unit required by regulatory authorities for stating vitamin E potency on labels. It recognizes that handedness affects potency, just as one of a person's hands is stronger than the other.

One milligram of the synthetic vitamin E, dl-Alpha tocopheryl acetate, is equal to one International Unit of vitamin E. The two letters "d" and "l" in combination is a chemist's way of indicating that the molecules are built on both the left-handed and right-handed pattern.

The same National Formulary goes on to specify that one milligram of d-Alpha tocopheryl acetate equals 1.36 International Units (36% more).

It takes careful reading to note the difference in those chemical names:

dl-Alpha tocopheryl acetate

d-Alpha tocopheryl acetate

That small "l" results in a lower potency. When it is NOT there you are being informed that the molecules have indeed all been assembled nature's way.

This doesn't mean that it is necessarily a better nutrient. It just means that less of it is required to do whatever essential biochemical job is to be done in your body by the vitamin E. It doesn't say that the chemist hasn't tinkered with the molecule nature made. The absence of that little "l" doesn't even prove that nature actually built those particular molecules, although actually building them in a laboratory from their constituent atoms would have been exorbitantly expensive. If the consumer wants "d" rather than "dl" it is far more practical to let nature do the molecule building out in the field where she makes vegetable oil.

If, for reasons of your own, you prefer the naturally

157

derived form of vitamin E, just look at the label carefully. Find that little "d" that goes with tocopheryl (sometimes it's tocopherol). Be sure that it applies to all the vitamin E in the product. If there is a little "l" after the little "d," there is vitamin E in it that did not start out from natural vegetable oils, whatever else may be stated about natural oils contained.

Not that synthetic vitamin E would harm you.

It's just that you have a right to know.

CHAPTER 16

Food Technologists Assess Vitamin E

"VITAMIN E" IS the title of an article in *Nutrition Reviews* for February, 1977. It was written by the Institute of Food Technologists Expert Panel on Food Safety and Nutrition and the Committee on Public Information. It purports to be a summary of the situation in regard to vitamin E.

It begins with these words, "Few topics are so charged with emotion, claims and counterclaims as is that of vitamin E and its benefits." True, they say, there are some scattered researchers who feel, as one California expert does, that "the more research is done on the substance, the more intriguing its appears. Thus there is the nagging suspicion that there is a very important use for the vitamin and we are just not smart enough to see it." This was said by Dr. A. L. Tappel in 1973.

The article goes on to tell the history of vitamin E, the food sources, the chance of losing some vitamin E in processing (deep fat frying of frozen foods, for example) and the recommended dietary allowance which is 12 to 15 milligrams daily for adults.

So, say this group of food technologists, "The facts, then, that vitamin E is commonly available, is stored in tissues throughout the body and is turned over very slowly in the body essentially preclude the existence of diseases which are truly the result of a vitamin E deficiency in man."

True, they go on, such deficiencies can be produced easily in experimental animals and birds. But this has no relevance for human beings. (It doesn't? Then why do researchers test and observe animals and birds and then apply their findings to human beings?) This is the customary method of research in all modern laboratories.

There are three circumstances, says the article, in which vitamin E is helpful. In a certain kind of anemia in premature infants essential vitamin E is not transferred across the placenta to the developing infant, so these children must be given vitamin E right from birth. In addition, human milk is very rich in vitamin E, but cow's milk is not. Commercial formulas often contain medicinal iron which destroys any vitamin E present and the unsaturated fats used in many infant formulas raise the baby's need for vitamin E.

Passing casually over this staggering array of evidence of vitamin E deficiency right from the moment of birth in most modern babies, the article goes on to say that, of course, anybody who may have difficulty dealing with the fats in their food (like post-surgery patients with part of their stomachs removed, people with cystic fibrosis, jaundice, pancreatic insufficiency or sprue, a chronic disease characterized by diarrhea and ulceration of the mucous membrane of the digestive tract), any or all of these people will of course be deficient in vitamin E and all the other fat-soluble vitamins (vitamins A, D and K) as well. How many Americans do you suppose the above categories cover? Half a million? A million? Two million?

But never mind, says the article in essence, there is only one other condition in which it has been proven by doubleblind studies that vitamin E "works." That is intermittent claudication, which is a circulatory ailment in which leg arteries are so clogged with deposits that the patient cannot walk more than a few feet without suffering agonizing pain in the legs. They quote two references to experiments in which this condition was cured with 400 milligrams of vitamin E daily over a period of three months. They do not mention that no other therapy for this condition exists nor do they point out that, since this one circulatory condition can be so easily cured by vitamin E, doesn't it seem likely that other circulatory problems might benefit from the vitamin?

It's true, the article continues, vitamin E functions as an antioxidant, which means that it prevents fats from becoming rancid, both in food and in body cells. Certain fats appear to degenerate and turn rancid in older folks. It appears that vitamin E can prevent this process. And it appears that vitamin E can and does protect vitamin A from destruction. But then how important is all this? they ask in essence. Well, older people just might believe that it's very important, don't you think?

The article goes on to say that vitamin E appears to neutralize "free radicals" which may be the basic cause of aging, but then this theory "is in a very early state" so we shouldn't be very concerned with it. Of course, Dr. Tappel tested a group of mice with quite large amounts of vitamin E added to their highly nutritious diets and found that the vitamin does indeed cut in half the incidence of "age spots" or "liver spots" in tissues, which usually indicate aging. But then the mice didn't live any longer than expected, so this experiment didn't really prove very much, says the article.

And how about cancer? Well, it's true that vitamin E provides absolute protection against several of the most toxic air pollutants in urban air, turning out to be "the most important defensive system against oxidant insult to lungs from air pollution." And, says the article, many of the basic features of these animal tests are similar to conditions affecting some humans. It thus appears warranted to "speculate about the application of these results to humans."

Did you ever read such an irresponsible statement from

a supposedly scientific body? In general they are saying, "Yes, folks, you can probably save yourself from dying of lung cancer caused by air pollution by taking some vitamin E, but of course you shouldn't do this until we scientists have had time to speculate about it, mull it over and see if it is 'warranted'."

Is vitamin E likely to cause trouble in massive doses? Well, nobody has ever reported any such thing, but then you can't be too sure, say these food technologists who are employed full-time, remember, by food and chemical companies to develop chemicals for food which will go out, all but completely untested for toxicity, to hundreds of millions of people to be eaten every day for the rest of their natural lives. And they are worrying here about a harmless vitamin which, so far, has brought benefit to millions of people and animals.

Most preposterous of all the assumptions and assertions made in the article is the statement that "vitamin E is so prevalent in common foods" that we need not make any special efforts to get it. Food technologists are the very people who have done everything possible to remove vitamin E from our food supply by refining flour and cereals, then bleaching the flour with chlorine which destroys finally any shred of vitamin E that might be left after the refining.

They are fully aware of this nutritional outrage. Yet they continue to insist that modern American diets are just loaded with vitamin E when they themselves have been most responsible for removing it from daily food. They are also fully aware of surveys and analyses which have been done which demonstrate clearly that the American diet, from baby's formulas right on to the toast and tea meals of our older folks, is so deficient in vitamin E that there is hardly a chance that anybody, even those who go out of their way to eat nutritionally sound meals, will ever get even the basic 12 to 15 milligrams daily which is officially recommended.

Suggested Further Reading

Adams, Ruth, *The Complete Home Guide to All the Vitamins*, Larchmont, 1976.

Adams Ruth and Frank Murray, *The New High Fiber Approach to Relieving Constipation Naturally*, Larchmont, 1977.

Cheraskin, E. and W. M. Ringsdorf, Jr., *New Hope for Incurable Diseases*, ARCO, 1971.

Clark, James W., E. Cheraskin and W. M. Ringsdorf, Jr., *Diet and the Periodontal Patient*, Charles C. Thomas, 1970.

Kalokerinos, Archie, *Every Second Child*, Thomas Nelson, 1974.

Passwater, Richard, *Supernutrition*, Simon and Schuster, 1975.

Passwater, Richard, *Supernutrition for Healthy Hearts*, Dial Press, 1977.

Shute, Evan V., *The Heart and Vitamin E*, Keats Publishing, 1976.

Shute Foundation for Medical Research, *Common Questions on Vitamin E and their Answers*, The Foundation, 1961.

Shute, Wilfrid E. and Harald Taub, *Vitamin E for Ailing and Healthy Hearts*, Pyramid, 1969.

Shute, Wilfrid E., *Complete Updated Vitamin E Book*, Keats Publishing, 1975.

Index

A

Adrenal Metabolic Research Society, 105, 106
Adriamycin, 23
Aging, 26, 40, 61, 68ff.
Agricultural and Food Chemistry, 11
Air pollution (smog), 34, 41, 42, 66, 70, 71, 77, 78, 81ff., 140
Alabama, University of, 141
Alcohol, alcoholism, 16, 41, 75
Allergies, 37, 97
American Academy of Dermatology, 124
American Chemical Society, 77
American Heart Association, 51
The American Journal of Clinical Nutrition, 6, 16, 36, 52, 61, 70, 95, 107, 115
American Journal of Diseases of Children, 105
American Journal of Obstetrics and Gynecology, 90, 112
American Medical Association, 46, 122
American Societies for Experimental Biology, 152
Amino acids, 21, 86, 105
Anemia, 41, 98, 109, 110, 111, 113, 114
Anfield, Dr. C., 98
Angina pectoris, 21, 55, 56, 58, 59, 61, 62, 90
Antibiotics, 41
Anti-coagulant drugs, 29, 33
Antioxidants, 78, 80, 81, 86, 99, 109, 115

Archives of Dermatology, 21, 125
Archives of Environmental Health, 82
Arkansas, University of, 22
Arteries, thrombosis in, 19
Arthritis, 18, 152
Aspirin, 32, 41
Athletes, 17, 31, 151
Atkins, Dr. Robert C., 63
The Australian Veterinarian, 22
Ayres, Dr. Samuel, Jr., 31

B

Babies, premature, 87ff., 108ff.
Baby foods, 116
Bacteria, 149
Barker, Dr. J. H., 39
Battelle-Northwest Institute, 84
Bed sores, 19, 118ff.
Bland, Dr. Jeffrey, 77
Blood clots, clotting, 16, 28, 32, 34, 41, 58, 66, 90
Blood sugar levels, 42, 43
Blood vessels, 25
Boggs, Dr. Thomas R., 115
Bottle-fed babies, 97, 116
Bran, 132
Breast cancer, 148ff.
Breast feeding, 97, 100
Breast milk, 100, 104, 110
Briggs, Michael and Maxine, 95
British Journal of Hematology, 26
British Journal of Nutrition, 12
British Medical Journal, 48, 49, 112, 114
Buerger's Disease, 19, 135ff.
Burns, 46, 72, 118ff.

164

C

Calcium, 29, 77
California Medicine, 62
California, University of, 42, 68, 71, 81, 91, 124, 137, 147
Calloway, Dr. Nathaniel C., 75
Canadian Family Physician, 59
Canadian Journal of Physiology and Pharmacology, 20, 59, 90
Canadian Medical Journal, 125
Cancer, 23, 24, 28, 34, 41, 73, 80, 85, 92, 148
Cathcart, Dr. Robert F., III, 30
Cells, human and animal, 68ff., 77, 81, 92, 149
Cereals, processed, 51, 52, 101
Chadd, Dr. M. A., 110
Chemical and Engineering News, 23, 84
Chen, Dr. L. H., 63
Cheraskin, Dr. E., 13, 141, 145
Chlorine, 26
Cholesterol, 10, 22, 50, 55, 56, 61, 63, 64, 65, 77, 138
Chromosomes, 80
Cincinnati, University of, Medical Center, 22
Circulation, circulatory problems, 16, 19, 20, 25, 32, 34, 54, 59, 60, 74, 95, 130, 150
Clark, Dr. James W., 145
Cleave, Dr. T. L., 48, 131
Cleveland Clinic, 149
Clinical Research, 18
Cohen, Dr. H. M., 62
Colorado State University, 151
Colostrum, 94, 97
Common Questions on Vitamin E and Their Answers, 64, 134
Consumer Bulletin, 99
Constipation, 131
Contraceptives (see "The Pill")
Cooley's Anemia, 25
Cornell Medical Index Questionnaire, 15
Cornell University, 152
Corn oil, 9

Coronary thrombosis, 56, 58
Cottonseed oil, 9
Cranston, Senator Alan, 96
Crib Death, 106, 107
Crib Death, 96ff.
Cumberland County College, 26

D

Davis, Dr. Karen C., 107, 115
DeLiz, Dr. A. J., 19
Dental Abstracts, 18, 138
Dental problems (see "Gums")
Dermolytic bullous dermatosis, 124
Diabetes, 19, 31, 42, 60, 65, 90, 122
Dicks-Bushnell, Dr. Martha, 107
Die Kapsel, 90
Diet and the Periodontal Patient, 145
Digestion, problems with, 7
Digitalis, 57
DiLuzio, Dr. D. N., 42
Diuretics, 41, 57, 75
Dodd, Dr. Harold, 130
Down's Syndrome, 93
Drury, Dr. Emma-Jane E., 11
Duke University, 34, 82

E

Eczema, 90, 130
Edema (swelling), 60, 86
Eggs, 50
Emphysema, 34
Environmental Research, 86
Enzymes, 73, 146, 149, 152
Epidermis bullosa, 127
Every Second Child, 102, 107
Executive Health, 29
Exercise, value of, 20, 61, 133
Eyes, problems with, 42, 74, 109, 113, 114

F

Farrell, Dr. Philip M., 36
Fats, animal, 48ff.
Fats, unhealthful, 42

Fats, unsaturated, 10, 12, 34, 84, 99, 108, 109, 110, 116, 138, 140, 149
Federal Trade Commission, 51
Federation Proceedings, 21
Fertility and Sterility, 87, 91
Fertility, infertility, 64, 87ff., 93
Fertilizers, commercial, 150, 151
Fisher, Dorothy, 122
Folic acid, 98, 111
Food and Drug Administration, 8, 150
Fortschiritte du Med., 59
Fraser, Dr. A. J., 110
Free radicals, 73

G

Gangrene, 19, 43, 120, 122, 135
Georgia, University of, 52
Gerloczy, Dr. F., 19, 136
Gieri, Dr. John G., 36
Goodson, Dr. J. Max, 137, 138
Graeber, Janet E., 108
Guidice, Dr. Del, 126
Gums, diseases of, 19, 137ff.
Gunther, Dr. Mavis, 97
Gynecol. Practique, 60

H

Hardening of the arteries, 20, 56, 60, 61, 90
Harris, Jan, 72
Headaches, 37
The Heart and Vitamin E, 67
Heart beat, irregular, 59
Heart disease, 22, 23, 32, 41, 42, 48ff., 136
Heart disease, prevention of, 64
Heart murmur, 55
Hemorrhages, 29, 33, 60, 86, 89, 99, 127
Hemorrhoids, 130
Herrick, J. B., 23
Herting, Dr. David C., 11
Hicks, Dr. B. S., 13
High blood pressure, 31, 34, 41, 55, 56, 65, 150

Hoffer, Dr. Abram, 27, 76
Homeostasis Quarterly, 105
Hormone drugs, 18, 24, 74
Horwitt, Dr. Max K., 32, 42
Hull, Mrs. Betty, 128
Huxley Institute for Biosocial Research, 74
Hypoglycemia (see "Low blood sugar")
Hypoglycemia Foundation, 105

I

Idaho, University of, 116
Immunization, of children, 102ff.
Infants, 96ff., 108ff.
Infections, 28, 97
Injuries, 28, 30
Institute of Food Technologists, 159
Insulin, 43, 90, 120, 122
Intermittent claudication, 20, 42, 110
International Academy of Preventive Medicine, 118
International Association of Bioinorganic Scientists, 147
International Journal of Vitamin Research, 110
International Units, 5, 6, 157
Iron, 77, 108, 110, 111, 113
Iron and vitamin E, 108
Itching, 74

J

Japanese Rheumatism Society, 25
Johnson, Dr. Lois, 113, 115
The Journal of Animal Science, 112
The Journal of Nutrition, 64
Journal of Oral Medicine, 142
The Journal of Pediatrics, 108
Journal of the American Dietetic Association, 13
The Journal of the American Geriatrics Society, 13
The Journal of the American

Medical Association, 30, 133
Journal of the American Podiatry Association, 134
Journal of the Canadian Medical Women's Association, 21
Journal of the Palacky University, 89
Journal of Vitaminology, 60, 128

K

Kalokerinos, Dr. Archie, 102
Keinholz, Dr. Eldon W., 151
Klenner, Dr. Fred, 103

L

La Leche League, 101, 117
The Lancet, 93, 97, 98, 130, 131, 132, 133, 151
Lardy, Dr. Henry, 105
Lattey, Dr. M., 59
Lecithin, 99, 100
Legs, leg cramps, 19, 20, 22, 25, 30, 37, 58, 110, 130ff., 135ff., 151
Liver, fatty, 60
Louisiana State University, 73
Low blood sugar, 105
Lungs, lung cells, 34, 82, 84, 85, 86, 99, 113
Lupus erythematosus, 128
Lupus Lifeline, 128

M

MacKenzie, Dr. John K., 42
Malnutrition, 77, 102
Marks, Dr. J., 109
Masai, 49
Massachusetts Institute of Technology, 84
McKay, Dr. D. G., 89
Medical Tribune, 17, 77
Medical World News, 18, 25, 113, 114
Medigraph Manual, 135
Memory, loss of, 20
Menopause, 60, 90

Menstruation, 90, 93
Mental and Elemental Nutrients, 146
Mental illness (see also "Schizophrenia"), 20, 126
Menzel, Dr. Daniel B., 34, 85
Mercury poisoning, 27
Methionine, 21, 86
Miami Heart Institute, 75
Michener, W. M., 125
Milk, 50
Milligrams, 5, 16, 157
Minamata Disease, 27
Minerva Ginecologia, 89
Minerals, trace, 8
Miscarriages, 89, 90
Money, Dr. F. C., 98
Montreal, University of, 72
Morris, Dr. Manford D., 22
Muscle weakness, 18, 22, 62
Muscular dystrophy, 22, 64
Myocardial infarction, 59

N

National Academy of Sciences, 5, 153
National Cancer Institute, 23, 85
National Formulary, 157
National Institutes of Health, 36, 87, 105
Nature, 99
Neuralgia, 21, 27
New England Journal of Medicine, 7, 61, 62
New Hope for Incurable Diseases, 145
New Mexico School of Medicine, University of, 125
New Scientist, 72
The New York Times, 26, 69, 105
Nitrogen oxide, nitrogen dioxide, 34, 82, 84, 85, 140
Nitroglycerin, 22, 56, 62
Novich, Dr. Max M., 18
Nuclear power plants, 28
Nutrition Reviews, 114, 159

O

Obesity, 60, 63, 65
Obstetrics and Gynecology, 89
Ochsner, Dr. Alton, 28
Olive oil, 9
Oregon, University of, 88
Overweight (see "Obesity")
Oxidants, 26, 71
Oxygen, 16, 27, 41, 66, 73, 75, 81, 90, 91, 98, 99, 109, 113, 115, 140
Oxygen therapy, 41, 114
Ozone, 34, 41, 82, 84, 86, 140

P

Packer, Dr. Lester, 40, 68, 81
Paley, Dr. George E., 135
Passwater, Dr. Richard, 53
Peanut oil, 9
Pennsylvania, University of, 113
Pfeiffer, Dr. Carl, 146
Phlebitis (see also "Thrombophlebitis"), 56, 58, 130, 134, 135
Phlebothrombosis, 28
Physiology, Chemistry and Physics, 64
The Pill, 41, 95
Polyunsaturated fatty acids, 138
Pregnancy, 21, 87ff., 130, 133
Premature babies (see "Babies, premature")
Prevention, 53
Proceedings of the Canadian Federation of Biologists Society, 59
Proceedings of the National Academy of Sciences, 80
Proceedings of the Workshop on Diet, Nutrition and Periodontal Disease, 138
Processed foods (see also "Cereals, processed"), 131ff., 138, 147
Prostaglandins, 137, 140
Prostatitis, 58

Protein, 98, 113, 142
Pryor, Dr. William A., 73
Psoriasis, 90
Pulmonary embolism, 34
Purpura (see "Hemorrhages")
Pyorrhea, 137ff.

Q

Quinine, 30

R

Radiation, 27, 73
Radiation Research, 27
Rancidity, 114, 115, 149
Raring, Richard H., 106
Recommended Daily Dietary Allowances, 5
Recommended Dietary Allowances, 5, 107
Rectal cramps, 31
Red blood cells, 16, 28, 33, 34, 77, 82, 112, 114, 139, 140
Rees, Dr. Rees B., 124
Respiratory Distress Syndrome, 99
Retinitis pigmentosa, 109
Retrolental fibroplasia, 99, 109, 113, 114, 115
Rheumatic heart disease, 25, 41, 64
Rheumatism, 24
Ringsdorf, Dr. W. M., Jr., 13, 145
Rinsho Derma, 27
Rosenthal, Herbert C., 135
Roy, Dr. R. M., 27
Royal College of Physicians, England, 48

S

Saffioti, Dr. Umberto, 85
Safflower oil, 9
Sambura, 49
Samuelson, Robert J., 50
Scars, scar tissue, 16, 72, 118ff., 120
Schaffer, Dr. David, 115

Schizophrenia, 19, 77

Schrauzer, Dr. Gerhard, 147

Schwartz, Herbert, 26

Science, 91

Science News, 81, 137

Scientific American, 73

Scott, Dr. Milton L., 152

Selenium, 9, 23, 98, 146ff.

Selenium, food sources of, 153

Selenium, amounts in soil and
    water, 149ff.

Selye, Dr. Hans, 72

Senility, 74, 75, 76

Sex organs, problems with, 74

Shamberger, Dr. Raymond, 149

Shingles, 21, 26

Shute, Dr. Evan, 15, 44, 61, 90,
    91, 94, 112, 118, 122, 136

Shute, Dr. Wilfrid, 72, 130

Shute Institute; Shute
    Foundation for Medical
    Research, 15, 27, 39, 64, 72,
    134

Skin, 37, 72

Skin and Allergy News, 124

Skin disorders, 19, 21, 60, 118ff.,
    124ff.

Smith, Dr. Bryan C., 88

Smith, Dr. E. B., 125

Smith, Dr. James R., 68, 81

Smoking (see also "Tobacco"),
    42, 61, 66, 77, 78, 104, 135

Society for the Protection of the
    Unborn Through Nutrition
    (SPUN), 101

Soderwall, Dr. A. L., 88

Soil, depletion of nutrients, 8

Soviet Academy of Medical
    Sciences, 17

Soybean oil, 9

St. Louis University School of
    Medicine, 32

Stamina, 17

Sterility (see also "Fertility,
    infertility"), 87, 90, 91

Steroid drugs, 17, 18, 24

Stillbirths, 21, 90

Strokes, 33, 95, 136

Sudden Infant Death Syndrome

(SIDS) (see "Crib Death")

Sugar, 41, 48, 52, 75, 105, 142,
    148

Sulfur, 146

The Summary, 16, 19, 39, 42, 44,
    61, 74, 90, 91, 93, 112, 122,
    127, 136

Supernutrition for Healthy Hearts,
    53

*Supernutrition: The Megavitamin
    Revolution,* 53

Surgery, 28, 29

T

Tapp, Dr. E., 98

Tappel, Dr. A. L., 42, 71, 159

Taub, Harald, 130

Texas, University of, 52, 74

Thalassemia, 113

Thrombophlebitis, 19, 112

Thyroid gland, 21, 60, 65

Tierarztliche Umschau, 63

Tobacco, 41

Toone, Dr. W. M., 61

Toronto Star, 39

*Toxicology and Applied
    Pharmacology,* 27

Tranquilizers, 41

Triglycerides, 61

Tulane University School of
    Medicine, 28

Turner, David, 41

U

Ulcers, 19, 43, 58, 90, 120, 122,
    126, 134

University College, London, 73

Unsaturated fats (see "Fats,
    unsaturated")

V

Varicose veins, 130ff.

Vegetarians, 154

Veterinary Medicine, 23

Viruses, 104, 149

Vitamin A, 33, 46, 61, 64, 77, 84,

85, 88, 91, 109
Vitamin B1, 77
Vitamin B3, 46, 76, 77
Vitamin B6, 77
Vitamin C, 29, 44, 46, 61, 77, 80, 86, 101, 122
Vitamin D, 33, 64, 77
Vitamin E, amount in average diet, 5, 12ff., 70
Vitamin E, amount in specified products, 9, 11
Vitamin E and iron, 108
Vitamin E and selenium, 146ff.
Vitamin E, as an antioxidant, 26
Vitamin E Content of Foods and Feeds for Human and Animal Consumption, 9
Vitamin E, foods containing, 45, 47, 101
Vitamin E for Ailing and Healthy Hearts, 130
Vitamin E, harmlessness of large doses, 36, 62, 141
Vitamin E, history of, 44
Vitamin E, loss from processing, 10ff., 33
Vitamin E, measurements in milligrams and International Units, 16
Vitamin E, natural vs. synthetic, 16, 155ff.
Vitamin E, need for, 15, 39, 138

Vitamin E, reason for deficiencies, 7, 41
Vitamin E, recommended daily dietary allowances, 5
Vitamin E, usefulness of, 16
Vitamin E, Wonder Worker of the '70's? 121
Vitamin K, 32, 64
Vitamins, absorption of, 16
Vitamins and Hormones, 109

W

Warfarin, 32
Washington Post, 50
Wheat germ, 17
Wheat, vitamin E content of, 9
Wheat germ oil, 9, 17, 88
Williams, Dr. Roger J., 52, 74
Willis, Dr. Charles E., 150
Wilson, Dr. H. D., 125
Wisconsin, University of, 75, 105
Wounds, 30, 72, 118ff.
Wrinkles, 72
Wyoming, University of, 9, 106

XYZ

X-rays, 28, 41, 77
Yale University, 113
Yellowlees, Dr. Walter, 49

Larchmont
Preventive Health Library

The Library will consist of the following books, issued as indicated. For quick reference, we have left off the full title of each book, which is "Improving Your Health with Vitamin A," etc.

1978

1. Vitamin A
2. Niacin (Vitamin B3)
3. Vitamin C
4. Vitamin E
5. Calcium and Phosphorus
6. Zinc

1979

7. Thiamine (B1) and Riboflavin (B2)
8. Pyridoxine (B6)
9. Iodine, Iron and Magnesium
10. Sodium and Potassium
11. Copper, Chromium and Selenium
12. Vitamin B12 and Folic Acid

1980

13. Vitamin D and Vitamin K
14. Pantothenic Acid
15. Biotin, Choline, Inositol and PABA
16. Protein and Amino Acids
17. Natural Foods
18. Other Trace Minerals

*The best books on health and
nutrition are from*

LARCHMONT BOOKS

—"**New High-Fiber Approach to Relieving Constipation
Naturally,**" by Adams and Murray; foreword by Sanford
O. Siegal, D.O., M.D.; 320 pages, $1.95

—"**Program Your Heart for Health,**" by Frank Murray;
foreword by Michael Walczak, M.D., introduction by E.
Cheraskin, M.D., D.M.D.; 368 pages, $2.95.

—"**Food for Beauty,**" by Helena Rubinstein; revised and
updated by Frank Murray, 256 pages, $1.95.

—"**Eating in Eden,**" by Ruth Adams, 224 pages, $1.75.

—"**Is Low Blood Sugar Making You a Nutritional
Cripple?**" by Ruth Adams and Frank Murray, 176 pages;
introduction by Robert C. Atkins, M.D.; $1.75.

—"**Beverages,**" by Adams and Murray, 288 pages, $1.75.

—"**Fighting Depression,**" by Harvey M. Ross, M.D.; 224
pages, $1.95.

—"**Health Foods,**" by Ruth Adams and Frank Murray,
foreword by S. Marshall Fram, M.D.; 352 pages, $2.25.

—"**Minerals: Kill or Cure?**" by Ruth Adams and Frank
Murray; foreword by Harvey M. Ross, M.D.; 368 pages,
$1.95.

—"**The Compleat Herbal,**" by Ben Charles Harris, 252
pages, $1.75.

___"**Lose Weight, Feel Great,**" by John Yudkin, M.D.; 224 pages, $1.75.

___"**The Good Seeds, the Rich Grains, the Hardy Nuts for a Healthier, Happier Life,**" by Adams and Murray; foreword by Neil Stamford Painter, M.D.; 304 pages, $1.75.

___"**Megavitamin Therapy,**" by Adams and Murray, foreword by David Hawkins, M.D.; introduction by Abram Hoffer, M.D.; 288 pages, $1.95.

___"**Body, Mind and the B Vitamins,**" by Adams and Murray, foreword by Abram Hoffer, M.D.; 320 pages, $1.95.

___"**The Complete Home Guide to All the Vitamins,**" by Ruth Adams, foreword by E. Cheraskin, M.D.; 432 pages, $2.50.

___"**Almonds to Zoybeans,**" by "Mothey" Parsons, 192 pages, $1.50.

___"**Vitamin C, the Powerhouse Vitamin, Conquers More than Just Colds,**" by Adams and Murray, foreword by Frederick R. Klenner, M.D.; 192 pages, $1.50.

___"**Vitamin E, Wonder Worker of the '70's?**" by Adams and Murray, foreword by Evan V. Shute, M.D.; 192 pages, $1.25.

**Read What the Experts Say
About Larchmont Books!**

Body, Mind and the B Vitamins

"I feel that "Body, Mind and the B Vitamins" is an excellent, informative book. I recommend everyone buy two copies; one for home and one to give to their physician."—*Harvey M. Ross, M.D., Los Angeles, Calif.*

Program Your Heart for Health

"What is unique about this book is that the tremendous body of fascinating information has been neatly distilled so that the problems and the solutions are quite clear. . . . (This book) will be around for a long time . . . so long as health continues to be the fastest growing failing business in the United States and so long as it is not recognized that the medical problem is not—medical but social."—*E. Cheraskin, M.D., D.M.D., Birmingham, Ala.*

"If more people were to read books such as this one and were to institute preventive medical programs early in life, the mortality in heart disease would drop precipitously as well as in our other serious medical problems."—*Irwin Stone, Ph.D., San Jose, Calif.*

"Program Your Heart for Health" contains a wealth of data. I plan to make use of it many times."—*J. Rinse, Ph.D., East Dorset, Vt.*